Other Titles by Christina Maria Gadar

For Students:

Pilates:
An Interactive Workbook

Pilates: An Interactive Workbook,
Wunda Chair Edition

For Teachers:

Pilates for Children:
Making Pilates Safe and Fun for Kids

For Children and Those Who Are Young at Heart:

Discovering Joe Pilates:
A Whimsical Exploration of Joe's Inventions

Coming Up:

The Pilates Animals Workout:
Exercise That Helps You Feel as Fit as an Animal

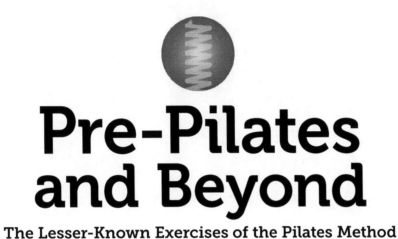

Pre-Pilates and Beyond

The Lesser-Known Exercises of the Pilates Method

Pre-Pilates and Beyond

The Lesser-Known Exercises of the Pilates Method

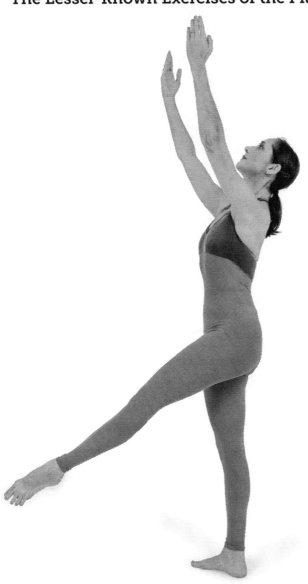

Christina Maria Gadar

2nd Generation Certified Pilates Teacher

Gadar, Christina Maria.
Pre-Pilates and beyond: the lesser-known exercises of the pilates method. /Christina Maria Gadar
ISBN: 978-1-7337864-1-6

Photography: Max Kelly
Interior Book Design: Yael Rotstein Campbell
Cover Design: Max Kelly
Model: Christina Maria Gadar
Pilates Mat: Gratz Industries

This book is for educational purposes only and is not intended to replace learning Pilates from a certified Pilates teacher. The author and Gadar Inc. d/b/a Gadar Pilates disclaims any and all liability for any adverse effects arising from the use or application of the information shown in this book.

To order more copies of *Pre-Pilates and Beyond*, visit:
www.PilatesPersonalTraining.com

Dedication

For my sister Denise and my tio Hamilton for their love and encouragement.

And for Joe Pilates, whose method of mind-body-spirit development has stood the test of time.

Acknowledgments

First and foremost, I must thank my ballet coach, premier danseur Fernando Bujones and my Pilates mentor, Romana Kryzanowska. My life has not been the same without their physical presence, but I will never forget the way they taught me, and the way they lived their lives to the fullest. Through teaching and writing, I hope to educate people about the importance of moving the body mindfully, as taught to me by Fernando, and the importance of preserving the integrity of Joseph Pilates' original vision of physical and mental conditioning, as taught to me by Romana.

In addition to working extensively with Fernando and Romana, I was blessed with the opportunity to study privately with two other pioneers in the field of movement, Hilary Cartwright and Igor Burdenko. When I was a teenager, Hilary taught me weekly body conditioning lessons at White Cloud Studio in New York. The exercise method I learned from Hilary is now known as the Gyrotonic® Method. Like Romana, she worked directly with the creator of the Method she taught. As the founder of the Burdenko Method in Massachusetts, Igor helped me recover from a broken leg and sprained ankle when I was dancing professionally. In addition to his land-based exercises, he developed exercises done in the pool that use the support and resistance of the water. Like Joe Pilates, Igor is an innovator and a genius of body movement. Hilary and Igor taught me that healing movement should not be painful, and that the power of positive thinking has a positive effect on the body.

I would also like to thank all my ballet teachers and Pilates teachers with whom I have studied. From the age of seven, I have studied with teachers who specialize in movement and each one has enhanced my understanding of the body as it moves through space. I consider it a privilege to be the recipient of their knowledge. **Please remember that this book is meant only for those who are already students of a certified Pilates teacher. Pilates *cannot* be learned from a book or a video – *only* from a teacher.**

This book would not exist without the expertise of Judith Rock, Max Kelly, and Yael Rotstein Campbell. Judith's passion for words makes her the ideal person to edit my books. Max is always patient and focused in our photo shoots and his beautiful book cover designs always exceed my expectations. I am grateful for Yael's knowledge, creativity, and meticulous eye for detail. She is the perfect person to design my books' interior layouts.

A special thank you goes to my students, who asked for this book, generously advised me on it, and waited for it with anxious anticipation. The fact that they want to study and practice Pilates on their own makes me feel validated as a teacher.

Finally, I must thank my family for their continued love and support. My mother, husband, children, uncle, sister, nephews and my many pets keep my life balanced and make it possible for me to pursue my dreams.

Contents

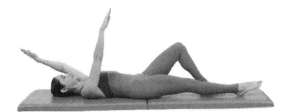

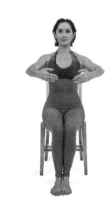

p. 1 INTRODUCTION

p. 3 HOW TO USE THIS WORKBOOK

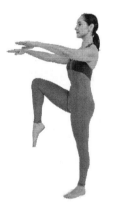

p. 4 PRE-PILATES EXERCISES

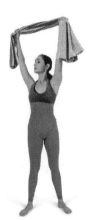

p. 63 WAKE-UP EXERCISES

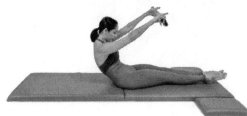

p. **71** BASIC MATWORK WITH A TOWEL

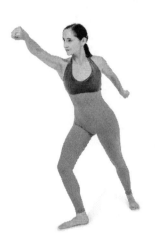

p. **82** JOE'S ARCHIVAL ROUTINE

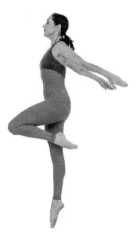

p. **103** ROMANA'S STANDING EXERCISES

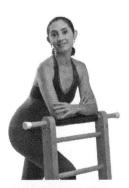

p. **112** ABOUT THE AUTHOR

Introduction

**"Physical fitness can neither be acquired
by wishful thinking nor by outright purchase."**

Joe Pilates in *Return to Life Through Contrology,* 1945

I became a Pilates teacher after a professional dancing career, and because I was trained to make movement look effortless, some of my Pilates students and colleagues are surprised when I tell them that I have had to work very hard to master certain Pilates skills. They seem especially surprised when they discover that, like them, I have aches and pains.

Maintaining my level of dancing onstage required a lot more effort outside the ballet studio in the last few years of my dance career. Pilates lessons, acupuncture treatments, and massage therapy were no longer optional, they were necessities. Twenty years later, some of my old dance injuries have resurfaced and some new injuries in what used to be healthy body parts have emerged. I view my experience as a dancer as a microcosm for life, with those last few years of dancing serving as a preview of what it can be like to cope with an aging body.

I sincerely believe that movement, and Pilates in particular, has curative powers. To stay healthy, you have to stay active, but at times, you have to let go of your ego and modify or even discontinue some of the activities that once came easily to you. One of the beautiful qualities of the Pilates Method is that it can be adjusted to fit your current situation, regardless of your experience, age, or health. A Pre-Pilates exercise aimed at increasing the range of movement in your neck can be just as exhilarating as a Standing Pilates exercise in which you skip across the room like a child. Pilates has been described as poetry in motion, and there is definitely an artistic component in doing the work, but beyond that, it is designed to help you enjoy your day-to-day life.

I discovered my love for the Pilates exercises in this book when I was writing *Pilates for Children: Making Pilates Safe and Fun for Kids*. In addition to teaching children exercises on the Pilates equipment, I wanted to offer options for teaching children in settings outside the studio, where Pilates equipment is not available. As I wrote about Pre-Pilates, Towel Exercises, and Standing Pilates, I began to incorporate these lesser-known movements into the lesson plans of my adult students. The response was very positive. Not only did they love these more obscure Pilates exercises, but they wanted to practice them on their own at home as well. I wrote *Pre-Pilates and Beyond: The Lesser-Known Exercises of the Pilates Method* for those who want a reference to these valuable exercises which, combined with the Matwork and the apparatus-work, make up the full spectrum of the Pilates Method.

WORK CITED

Pilates, Joseph H. *Return to Life Through Contrology*. 1945. The Christopher
   Publishing House, 1960.

How to Use This Book

No Pilates book can reveal the depth of practice necessary to achieve an understanding of the Method's true essence. **The only way to truly learn Pilates is to feel it in your own body with the guidance of a certified Pilates teacher.** But once you have an instructor, practicing Pilates at home on your own is also an important element in taking ownership of your workout and making the most of the time and money you invest in your lessons. **It is important to remember that you *never* perform any exercise on your own unless you have already practiced it in the studio with your instructor.**

The main areas covered in this book are Pre-Pilates Exercises, Towel Exercises, and Standing Pilates Exercises. These three groupings are further divided into five chapters. Within each chapter, the exercises are presented in an order that gradually increases in intensity.

The first chapter covers the Pre-Pilates Exercises. These exercises are divided into sections that focus on specific parts of the body, from the bottoms of the feet, all the way up to the top of the head. Each section also includes suggestions on how to progress to more advanced Pilates exercises that work the same body part. There is no specific order to the Pre-Pilates routine. Choose the Pre-Pilates exercises that target the areas of your body that need to be addressed.

The movements that make up the Towel Exercises are divided into two chapters: the Wake-Up Exercises and the Basic Matwork with a Towel. The Wake-Up Exercises are performed standing and do not require much space, just a bath towel held between the hands. The Wake-Up Exercises can be performed in their entirety or you can focus on individual exercises from the routine. If you have enough space to put your bath towel on the floor, you have enough room to practice your Basic Matwork. Incorporating the use of a hand towel in the Matwork can deepen stretches and provide additional support. It is recommended that the Matwork be done in the order presented, omitting any exercises that are not a good fit for your body.

The movements that make up the Standing Pilates Exercises are divided into two chapters: Joe's Archival Routine and Romana's Standing Exercises. The Standing Pilates exercises are more rigorous than the exercises presented in the other chapters. Depending on your individual needs, you can perform a single Standing Pilates exercise at the end of your home-based routine, or perform a group of standing exercises for a more intense workout. The sequences presented in the Standing Pilates chapters are very similar to the sequences used by Joe and Romana.

Pre-Pilates and Beyond has something for everyone. Use it together with my first book, *Pilates: An Interactive Workbook*, to create a well-rounded home-based routine that will improve your sense of autonomy and inspire you to assemble creative workouts tailored to your body.

Pre-Pilates

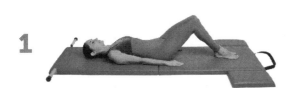

1

p. 10   BREATHING

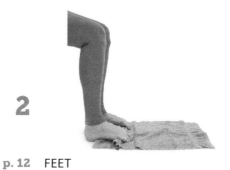

2

p. 12   FEET

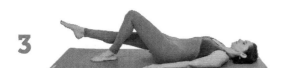

3

p. 22   KNEES

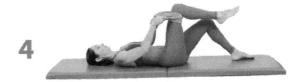

4

p. 24   HIPS

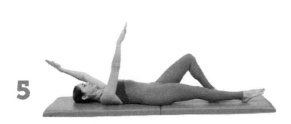

5

p.27   BACK

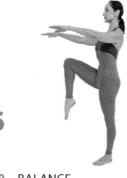

6

p.30   BALANCE

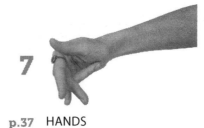

7

p.37   HANDS

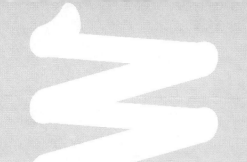

8

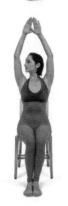

p. 42 ARMS

9

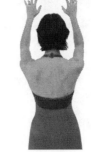

p. 47 SHOULDERS

10

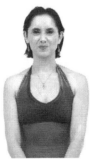
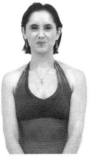

p. 52 NECK

11

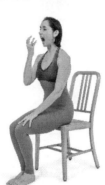

p. 58 JAW

12

p. 59 NOSE

13

p. 60 EYES

14

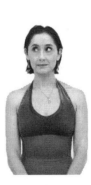

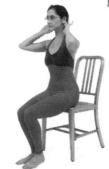

p. 61 EARS

Pre-Pilates

CONTENTS:

PRE-PILATES FOR BREATHING:
10   NASAL BREATHING

GOING BEYOND PRE-PILATES FOR BREATHING:
11   BREATHING DEVICE EXERCISE

PRE-PILATES FOR THE FEET:
12   SPREAD YOUR TOES
12   LIFT ONE TOE AT A TIME
12   WRITE THE ALPHABET WITH YOUR TOES
12   PICK UP A MARBLE
13   PICK UP A PENCIL
13   WALK A TIGHTROPE
13   TRACE THE FEET
14   TOE TAPPING
14   TOWEL FOOTWORK SITTING

GOING BEYOND PRE-PILATES FOR THE FEET:
15   RUBBER BAND EXERCISES
19   FOOTWORK STANDING
20   PRESSURE POINTS
21   FOOT MASSAGE

PRE-PILATES FOR THE KNEES:
22   LEG RAISES
23   TV EXERCISES

GOING BEYOND PRE-PILATES FOR THE KNEES:
24   SIDE LEG KICKS: FRONT/BACK
24   BRIDGE

PRE-PILATES FOR THE HIPS:
25   TOWEL UNDER THE THIGH
25   PRESSURE ON THE THIGHS
26   BRIDGE

GOING BEYOND PRE-PILATES FOR THE HIPS:
27   ONE LEG BALANCE
27   SINGLE LEG CIRCLES

PRE-PILATES FOR THE BACK:
27   HUG KNEE(S) TO CHEST
28   MOVING THE LIMBS AWAY FROM THE CENTER
29   LEG RAISES

GOING BEYOND PRE-PILATES FOR THE BACK:
29   HAMSTRING STRETCH
29   MAGIC CIRCLE ARMS
30   MAGIC CIRCLE LEGS

PRE-PILATES FOR BALANCE:
31   MARCHING
32   GLIDING STEP
33   GOOSE STEP

GOING BEYOND PRE-PILATES FOR BALANCE:
34   PILATES LUNGES
35   GOING UP FRONT WITH A LOW STOOL
36   LEG PUSH DOWN WITH A CHAIR FRAME
37   ONE LEG BALANCE
37   TREE STANDING

PRE-PILATES FOR THE HANDS:
37   SPREAD THE FINGERS
37   LIFT ONE FINGER AT A TIME
38   FINGER FLICKS
38   WRIST CURLS
39   WRIST TWIRLS/FLOREO
40   CASTANETS

GOING BEYOND PRE-PILATES FOR THE HANDS:
41   HAIR TIE EXERCISE
42   SAND BAG MOVEMENT WITH A ROLLING PIN

PRE-PILATES FOR THE ARMS:
43   SHAKING OUT THE ARMS
43   HUG WITH FISTS

GOING BEYOND PRE-PILATES FOR THE ARMS:

44   WALL SERIES: PEEL DOWN

45   STANDING WEIGHTS SERIES: STANDING CURLS

46   MAGIC CIRCLE ARM SERIES: ARMS IN FRONT AND BEHIND

46   JOE'S ARCHIVAL STANDING ARM EXERCISES

PRE-PILATES FOR THE SHOULDERS:

47   SHRUGS

48   SHOULDER ROLLS

48   SPIDER

GOING BEYOND PRE-PILATES FOR THE SHOULDERS:

49   PILATES PUSH-UPS ON THE WALL

50   PILATES PUSH-UPS ON THE FLOOR

51   L-SHAPE AGAINST THE WALL

52   WAKE-UP EXERCISES FOR THE UPPER BODY

52   CARTWHEELS

PRE-PILATES FOR THE NECK:

53   NOSE CIRCLES AND NECK SEMI-CIRCLES

53   NECK ROTATION

54   EAR TO SHOULDER

GOING BEYOND PRE-PILATES FOR THE NECK:

55   ASSISTED NECK STRETCH WITH THE TOWEL

55   MAGIC CIRCLE NECK EXERCISES WITH THE HANDS

57   CHEST EXPANSION

PRE-PILATES FOR THE JAW:

58   YAWN/BITE AN APPLE

PRE-PILATES FOR THE NOSE:

59   WIGGLE THE TIP OF THE NOSE

PRE-PILATES FOR THE EYES:

60   EYE CIRCLES

PRE-PILATES FOR THE EARS:

61   WIGGLE THE EARS

PRE-PILATES

"I give people homework, like exercises to do in bed before you even put your feet on the floor in the morning. We don't pop 'em into a class and command them to do a hundred sit-ups!"
Romana Kryzanowska in an interview with *TIME*.

INTRODUCTION

Even among Pilates professionals, the exercises in this chapter are a bit unfamiliar and the umbrella terms used to describe them can be confusing. Part of the confusion about the name comes from the fact that these exercises have many applications. When I started my Pilates apprenticeship, they were introduced as "Exercises for Injuries" because they are often given to students who need to work with specific parts of the body that are weak, tight, and/or recovering from injury. Later in my apprenticeship, I discovered that these exercises also give teachers a safe way to assess the strength and mobility of a new student who might not be ready to go into the traditional Pilates routine on the Reformer and Mat. That was when I heard them called "Pre-Pilates."

I learned the vast majority of the exercises presented in this chapter directly from Romana. But she didn't categorize them with a blanket term. She referred to some of them as "Wake-Up Exercises" because they are gentle enough to perform in the morning: exercises for the eyes, nose, ears, jaw, neck, and arms. Romana referred to other exercises as "TV Exercises" because they were simple enough to do at home while sitting in front of the television. Romana also taught "Exercises for Businessmen," so that her students who spent a lot of time on the road could stay strong and limber while away from the studio. Using just a towel, these students learned to stretch and strengthen their muscles while standing in a relatively small amount of space, the equivalent of a small hotel bathroom. I have put the "Exercises for Businessmen" in the next chapter called Wake-Up Exercises because they are more challenging than the exercises in this chapter.

To add to the confusion, Romana often said that there is no such thing as "Pre-Pilates." One of my master teachers told me that Romana disliked the term "Pre-Pilates" because she felt that the exercises did not represent Joe's original work. They may have originated with another former student of Joe Pilates, Eve Gentry. According to this master teacher, Romana felt that the Method as Joe taught it was enough on its own, and that these exercises were to be regarded as homework. Romana wanted her students to *move* in the studio, and the exercises in this chapter are static in comparison to the traditional Pilates exercises as Joe and Romana taught them. Other master Pilates teachers, also trained by Romana, believe that calling these exercises "Pre-Pilates" does not give them the recognition they deserve. Though they focus on single body parts, these exercises retain the integrity of the Pilates philosophy because the movement still initiates from the powerhouse.

For simplicity, I have decided to use the term "Pre-Pilates" in this book, because it is the name most commonly given to this group of exercises. While the name we give these exercises can be debated, the fact remains that Romana saw the value of giving these exercises to many of her students. Pre-Pilates exercises provide teachers with a wealth of information about students and are appropriate for students to perform on their own as homework. There is a Pre-Pilates exercise for almost every body part, from the toes all the way up to the scalp.

In addition to the applications previously mentioned, the Pre-Pilates exercises are a good way to define the body musculature and Pilates principles. Educating yourself about the way your muscles should move can help you avoid bad habits down the road. Through your practice of the Pre-Pilates exercises, you will learn that your powerhouse muscles should be engaged in order to isolate and move a specific body part. In the Pilates Method, you either create your own resistance or work with external resistance. The resistance helps you develop opposing lines of energy in your body. Learning to initiate these exercises from your powerhouse muscles will teach you to rely on your muscles and not your joints to do the work.

In time, you will notice that moving your body with a Pilates mindset will help you achieve correct body alignment and use less energy as your movements become more efficient. This is a connection that will help you in both the Pilates studio and in daily activities outside the studio.

The Pre-Pilates moves can be executed in various postures. Lying face up on a mat is the easiest of the postures because it provides the most body support. Seated exercises offer an added challenge, especially when performed while seated on the edge of a chair without leaning on the seatback. Standing is the most challenging position in which to execute an exercise, especially when performed without the back support of a wall, because the full body weight is on the legs.

Pre-Pilates exercises have value because we use them to recover from injuries and to prevent future injuries. I chose to personalize each of the introductions in this chapter to remind readers that, despite appearances, everyone has aches and pains. This chapter focuses on exercises I learned directly from Romana and her hand-chosen master teachers. Your teacher may know other exercises that could also be placed in this grouping. The *Going Beyond Pre-Pilates* sections in this chapter suggest suitable progressions for students who are ready to move from the Pre-Pilates exercises into the more demanding exercises from the traditional Pilates Method.

NOTE ABOUT GETTING TO THE FLOOR

Using a minimum of motion to create the maximum effect is one of the goals in Pilates. This idea is referred to as the Pilates principle of Flow. To transition with ease from standing to sitting, and sitting to standing, one should activate the other Pilates principles of Control, Centering, Concentration, Precision, and Breath.

Moving efficiently from standing to sitting on the floor will keep you safe and conserve your energy for the exercise. Crossing the forearms and the feet to lower your seat to the floor, as is done at the start of the Matwork, is one way to go from standing to sitting **(Photos A-D)**. But if deep knee bends are not a safe choice for your body, place your hands on the floor and swivel on the balls of your feet as you take a seat on the floor **(Photos E-H)**. To stand without putting any pressure on your knees, bend your legs **(Photo H)** and cross one foot over the other, rotate from your waist and put your hands on the floor to the side of the body that matches your front foot **(Photo G)**. Then swivel on the balls of your feet as you push your hands into the floor and lift your seat **(Photos F and E)**.

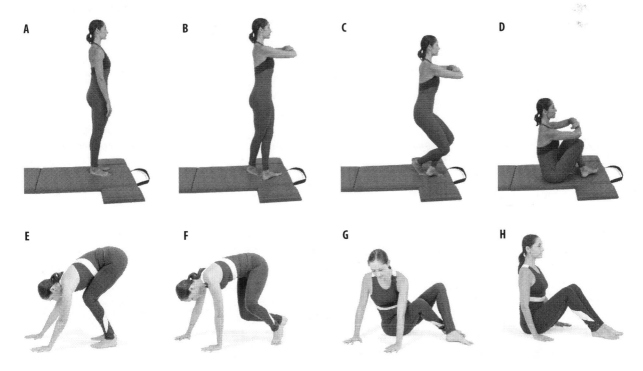

PRE-PILATES FOR BREATHING

INTRODUCTION

When I was in the middle of my Pilates apprenticeship, one of my grandmaster teachers challenged me to do the entire Reformer routine breathing only through my nose. She explained that the ideal breathing in Pilates is nasal breathing. Later, I learned that Joe Pilates drew much of his inspiration for the Contrology exercises from observing animals. While observing the way animals breathe during their waking hours and while they sleep, it is evident that most of them breathe through the nose and not the mouth. Breathing through the mouth usually indicates congestion or some other difficulty. In people, nasal congestion or a deviated septum can lead to breathing through the mouth. Specific issues aside, most animals will only breathe through their mouths when they need to regulate their temperatures by panting. Otherwise, they breathe as nature intended, through their noses.

When asked about the timing of the in-breath and out-breath in exercises that don't typically focus on breathing, Romana often said, "You don't tell a horse how to breathe, he just breathes." She wanted her students to put the focus on the powerhouse muscles and trust that the body would naturally fall into the correct breathing rhythm. It is worth noting that horses typically breathe through their nostrils. They only breathe through their mouths if they have an injury or an issue with the soft palate that separates the mouth from the nasal passages.

NASAL BREATHING

Getting Started

Sit in a comfortable position and alternate breathing in through one nostril and out through the other. To do this, press your right index finger on the outside of your right nostril to close it. Breathe in through your left nostril. Remove your right index finger and press your left index finger on the left nostril to close it. Breathe out through your right nostril. Complete the set with the in-breath through the right nostril and the out-breath through the left nostril. Perform 2-4 sets.

Why It's Beneficial

Nasal breathing is considered deeper than shallow breaths through the mouth. The nose acts as a natural humidifier and filtering system for the body. Nasal breathing humidifies the inhaled air, whereas breathing through the mouth creates dryness in the mouth and throat. Nasal breathing traps most particles, including dust, animal dander, and pollen, whereas breathing through the mouth permits more pollutants to enter the body. Since the nose tends to get blocked when breathing through the mouth, nasal breathing is especially important for people with allergies or asthma.

Note

If you have nasal congestion or a deviated septum, attempt nasal breathing for the in-breath only. With practice you might be able to add nasal breathing for the out-breaths, but if not, it is fine to breathe out through the mouth if you have nasal issues.

Eventually

To find the connection between deep breathing and the powerhouse, lie on your back with your legs bent, feet resting on the mat. Take a deep breath through your nose. As you breathe out through your nose, focus on images that deepen your powerhouse and help you anchor your back to the mat. Imagine that you are buttoning your bellybutton to the mat on each exhalation, or pretend that your back is spreading out on the mat like melted butter on each out-breath. Perform 3-5 sets of in-breaths and out-breaths. Try to increase the length of your exhalation each time. **Photo A**

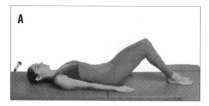

GOING BEYOND PRE-PILATES FOR BREATHING

BREATHING DEVICE EXERCISE

Note

The Breathing Device Exercise is the only Pilates exercise that is not done with nasal breathing. It is a good option for those with nasal issues.

Tips

You can use a pinwheel toy as a substitution for the Pilates Breathing Device. You can find instructions for making your own pinwheel on the Internet using a straw as the handle and a few pieces of paper held together with a push pin to form the wheel.

Getting Started

When first learning this exercise it is easy to get distracted by the breathing and forget to articulate the spine while bending forward. To emphasize the spinal articulation, perform this exercise with your back peeling away from a wall, rather than standing without back support.

With your back on the wall and your feet away from the wall, hold the handle of the pinwheel toy in front of your sternum. Take a deep breath and begin to exhale through your mouth as you peel one vertebra off the wall at a time. A longer exhalation is the goal. Once you truly have no more air left to breathe out, breathe in as you roll your spine back up onto the wall. Try to increase your exhalation on each repetition. Imagine that you are using one breath to blow out the candles on a birthday cake. Perform 3 times.

Why It's Beneficial

The Breathing Device Exercise develops breath control, empties the lungs, and aids in the articulation of the spine. Like the Peel Down from the Wall Series, it incorporates all the elements of a good exercise with which to end a lesson: breathing, spinal articulation, and inversion.

Using the Breathing Device while bending forward demonstrates and teaches how spinal articulation enhances breathing. As you roll forward, you might experience a moment when you cannot get the wheel to keep spinning, even though you are still exhaling. Then, as you bend forward a little more, you might be able to get more air out of the bottom of your lungs, which makes the wheel spin again. The combination of bending forward while breathing out is a concept that appears repeatedly in the Pilates syllabus.

Eventually

Once you are able to combine a deep exhalation with the deliberate articulation of your spine, you are ready to perform the same exercise standing away from the wall. When you do this exercise away from the wall, keep your weight forward on the balls of your feet while still pressing your heels into the floor. Perform 3 times. **Photos B-D**

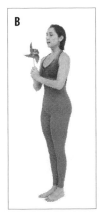
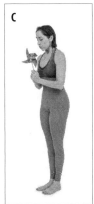
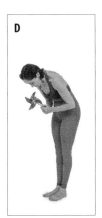

PRE-PILATES FOR THE FEET

INTRODUCTION

Joe Pilates believed that the feet are our foundation for a strong and healthy body. The fact that most people spend more time squeezing their feet into ill-fitting shoes than they do climbing trees barefoot has made our toes less flexible than our fingers. "The foot has evolved from its hand-like design to serve as a platform for the human body" (Biel 254). Joe Pilates recognized the importance of exercising the most used and abused part of our bodies. The fact that he begins the Reformer routine with the Footwork Series demonstrates the importance he placed on working the body from the ground up.

I was told innumerable times that I would never make it as a professional ballet dancer because my feet were too weak and inflexible. Although hard work and determination helped me prove my naysayers wrong, it was not without many set-backs. I broke both fifth metatarsals on four separate occasions, fractured my fibula, sprained my ankle, suffered from painful bunions, neuromas, plantar fasciitis, Achilles tendonitis, and bursitis. As a result of my struggle to get my feet strong and limber, I became very interested in exercises designed to improve foot alignment, mobility, and strength. Since discovering Pilates and incorporating it into my life, I have been able to keep my feet strong and flexible, and avoid painful arthritis in my feet, which is a common aftereffect among retired ballet dancers.

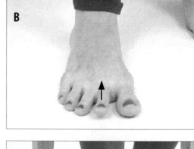

The following exercises can be done safely on your own. It is important to remember to engage your powerhouse muscles as you perform all foot exercises. Engaging the powerhouse muscles is the best way to attain correct form. For example, a student with fallen arches may benefit more from focusing on lifting her inner thighs rather than simply lifting her arches.

EXERCISE #1: SPREAD YOUR TOES

Alternate spreading your toes apart and drawing them together. It's a good way to counteract the time spent wearing shoes. **Photo A**

EXERCISE #2: LIFT ONE TOE AT A TIME

Lift one toe at a time off the floor. This is good for centering the focus. **Photo B**

EXERCISE #3: WRITE THE ALPHABET WITH YOUR TOES

Writing the alphabet with your toes improves the circulation in your feet and ankles. **Photo C**

EXERCISE #4: PICK UP A MARBLE

Pick up a marble with one toe at a time and deposit it in a container. **Photo D**

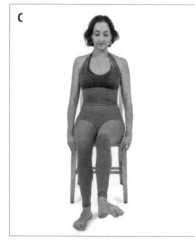

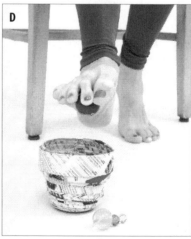

EXERCISE #5: PICK UP A PENCIL

Pick up a pencil with *all* your toes at once, not in between your toes. Despite being frustrating, it really works the feet. **Photo E**

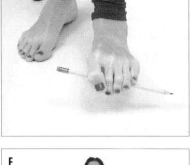

EXERCISE #6: WALK A TIGHTROPE

Walk an imaginary tightrope. This is good for balance control and for building strength around the metatarsals. **Photo F**

TRACE THE FEET

Getting Started

Stand on two feet with a piece of paper under one foot. Make sure that your weight is equally distributed on both feet as someone traces the outline of your foot on the paper. Take the drawing and make a dot on the ball of the foot near the two inside toes, a second dot on the ball of the foot near the two outside toes, and a third dot on the center of the heel. Looking at the two points on the ball of the foot explains why most of your weight should be toward the front of your foot and not back on your heel. Be sure to have someone trace your other foot to see if there is any discrepancy between the drawings.

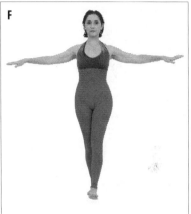

Now have someone trace your feet again while you focus on lifting through your waist and inner thighs, and engaging your seat muscles. With the powerhouse engaged, you will probably see a drawing that more closely represents the ideal positioning of the foot. This is an excellent visual aid for helping you see how engaging the powerhouse muscles affects the other muscles of your body. **Photo G**

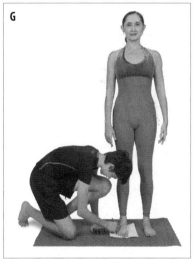

Why It's Beneficial

This exercise educates people about how to distribute the points of pressure in the foot. A Greek column begins with a strong base. To develop a strong base for your body, you need to keep your weight toward the balls of your feet with light pressure on your heels.

Tips

Practice standing correctly as you wait in line at the grocery store. Stand in the stance appropriate for your body, Pilates stance or with the feet parallel and slightly apart, and focus on pulling your bellybutton in and up as you shift your weight toward the balls of your feet. Make sure that you are not locking your knees or sinking into one of your hips.

Eventually

Standing correctly means that you are able to move instantly in any direction. Sitting into a hip or leaning back on your heels will make you waste time and energy readjusting your body weight in order to move. Stand on both feet and have someone give you a cue to move forward, backward, to the side, or on the diagonal. The less the reaction time between their cue and your movement, the more likely it is that you are distributing your weight efficiently on your feet.

TOE TAPPING

Getting Started

Sit near the edge of a chair with your feet on the floor and your arms extended down toward the floor. With your bellybutton pulling in and up, raise your heels off the floor and alternately tap the balls of your feet on the floor up to 30 times without leaning back. To finish, stretch your legs out in front of you. You will feel a tingling sensation in your feet. This exercise is similar to the Shaking Out the Arms Pre-Pilates exercise described later in this chapter. **Photo H**

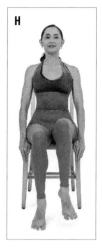

Why It's Beneficial

Toe Tapping improves the circulation in the feet. Because Toe Tapping is particularly good for the nerves in the feet, it is a wonderful exercise for people with neuropathy. Toe Tapping is also an excellent exercise for working the powerhouse muscles.

Tips

To tap into the powerhouse muscles, remember to sit tall and not lean back as you tap your toes.

Eventually

For an extra stretch in the feet, and for strengthening the wrists, you can put your hands on the front edge of your chair and lift your seat as you shift your weight onto the balls of your feet. Hold up to three seconds and release. Perform 1-3 times.

TOWEL FOOTWORK SITTING

Why It's Beneficial

The Towel Footwork Sitting will enhance the articulation of the feet and develop muscle strength. The Towel Footwork is especially beneficial to people with muscle imbalances in their feet. In Pilates, the arch is considered the powerhouse of the foot. The arch of the foot is made up of three distinct smaller arches. Using the three points of pressure from the foot tracing exercise, the medial longitudinal arch runs from the point at the ball of the foot near the two inside toes to the point at the center of the heel, the lateral longitudinal arch runs from the point at the ball of the foot near the two outside toes to the point at the center of the heel. The anterior transverse arch runs from the point near the big toe ball to the point near the little toe ball. The Towel Footwork works all three of these arches.

Getting Started

Sit near the edge of a chair. Your legs should be bent at a ninety-degree angle with the towel stretched out on the floor in front of you. With your feet and legs parallel and apart, position your toes on the bottom edge of the towel with your heels resting on the floor. The towel is not under your heels. Your bellybutton is lifted as you engage your seat muscles, and your inner thighs hug your midline.

Keep your heels on the floor and drag the towel toward you with the *balls* of both feet. To keep the work in the transverse arch, be sure that your toes remain long as your feet curl into a dome shape. Picking up marbles with the toes is not a good substitute for the Towel Footwork because it emphasizes curling the toes, as opposed to curling the foot. Imagine that you are making a parachute as you create the dome shape with your foot. After you pull the towel in as far as you can, lift the balls of your feet and your toes off the towel. Next, spread your toes in the air and extend them forward on the towel to complete the movement. **Photo I**

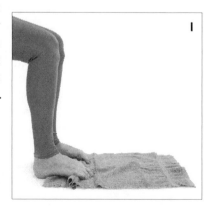

Once you have pulled the towel toward you as far as possible, push the towel away with your feet. Lift your toes off the towel, pull them toward your arch, and slide the balls of your feet on the towel with long toes to push the towel away from you. Imagine that you are at the beach, digging your toes through the sand.

This exercise can be performed with the feet moving in unison, and with one foot, then the other. When the feet alternate pulling on the towel, the motion will resemble the paws of a cat kneading a blanket. For fun, imagine that your feet are competing in a race to get the towel to the finish line. Perform 1 set, both pulling and pushing the towel, with the feet moving in unison, and another set with the feet taking turns.

Tips
This exercise requires a slick floor, such as tile or wood.

As you lift your arch off the floor to create a dome shape, make sure that you don't roll to the outer or inner side of your foot. You can avoid rolling the foot out of alignment as you go into the dome shape by letting a little daylight be visible along the outside edge of the foot, the lateral longitudinal arch, and the inside edge of the foot, the medial longitudinal arch. Imagine that you are making a tunnel, not a cave, as you dome your foot. There should be enough daylight at each end of the tunnel for a tiny snail to pass through.

Eventually
You can also turn the towel lengthwise and practice lateral movement with one foot at a time. This is a good variation for strengthening muscle imbalances in the feet. Start seated with your legs bent at ninety degrees. Position your right foot on the left edge of the towel. Lift the ball of your right foot and spread your toes as you rotate your ankle to the right side of the towel. Be sure to move from the ankle and not the hip. The knee does not open. Next, create a dome shape with your foot and slide the towel across the floor to your left while maintaining long toes and a lift in all of the arches of your foot.

After using your right foot to pull the towel to the left, repeat the movement with your right foot pushing the towel back to the right. After completing one set with the right foot, use the left foot to pull and push the towel. Perform 1 set on each foot. If one foot is noticeably weaker, perform an extra set with the weaker foot. If both feet are relatively equal in strength, but moving the towel in one of the two directions is noticeably harder, perform an extra set moving the towel in the direction that works the weaker side of the foot. For example, the outsides of my feet have always been weak and prone to injury, so I do extra sets pushing the towel away from my midline in order to build the strength around my fifth metatarsal.

GOING BEYOND PRE-PILATES FOR THE FEET

RUBBER BAND EXERCISES
Getting Started
Use a wide rubber band with medium to medium-light resistance. These rubber bands can be found in the produce section of your supermarket. Remove your socks and place the rubber band on your big toes. The rubber band should lie just below your toenails. If the rubber band is positioned at the base of the big toes it will not provide an adequate stretch in the larger joints of the big toes, the first metatarsal phalangeal joints. If the rubber band is placed too high, near the tip of the toes, it puts too much stress on the smaller joints of the big toes, the interphalangeal joints, and it is harder to keep the rubber band on the toes.

Sit near the edge of a chair with your legs bent at ninety degrees and your feet and legs parallel and apart. Just as the Reformer carriage supports the back in a supine position, the floor provides support for the feet in the introductory exercises with the rubber band. Keep your weight light on your feet so that you can move with more ease. It is very important that you look at the outside of your feet to determine if they are truly in a parallel position. The outsides of your heels should be in line with your little toes.

To prepare, engage your powerhouse muscles. Next, stretch the rubber band slightly, while your feet remain parallel and apart and your toes spread on the floor. The toes do not lift off the floor.

There are many toe exercise variations. Here are some of my favorites. I suggest concentrating on only one or two at a time.

VARIATION #1:
NOTE: This variation should be performed with a towel under your feet to help the feet remain parallel on the floor as the feet slide out and in.

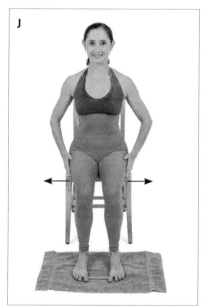

Sitting, with the rubber band on your big toes and your feet lightly touching the towel while remaining parallel and apart, press the outsides of your thighs away from each other as you slide the outsides of your feet away from your midline. The goal is to work the outer thighs and seat. The feeling is similar to the feeling of pushing the carriage out on the Side Splits exercise on the Reformer. Also, putting tension on the rubber band with the feet remaining in parallel allows the rubber band to give the big toe joints a nice stretch. This is a *small* movement, so be careful not to exaggerate the stretch. Press out on the rubber band for up to three seconds. Perform 3 times. **Photo J**

This exercise stretches the bunions and strengthens the outer thighs. The feet will remain parallel as they move apart. The movement of the feet will make the rubber band pull on the big toes.

VARIATION #2:
Sitting, with the rubber band on your big toes and your feet parallel and apart on the floor, press the outsides of your thighs away from each other as you rotate your ankles away from your midline. Even though the slight rotation happens at the ankles and not at the hips, be sure that the energy still originates from the powerhouse. Press out on the rubber band for up to three seconds. Perform 3 times with the feet moving in unison. **Photo K**

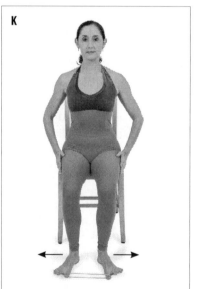

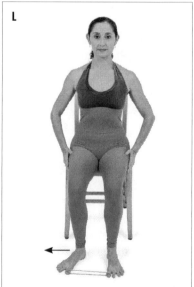

After three repetitions with both ankles rotating outward simultaneously, you can alternate rotating one ankle at a time away from your midline. Perform 2-4 times with the feet alternating. **Photo L**

This exercise strengthens the metatarsals. The ankles rotate away from each other as the big toes pull on the rubber band.

VARIATION #3:

Sitting, with the rubber band on your big toes and your feet parallel and apart on the floor, keep one foot on the floor as you flex your other foot. Your heel remains on the floor as the toes and sole of the foot lift away from the floor. Next, draw circles in the air with the big toe of your flexed foot. Perform 3 times and repeat 3 more circles in the reverse direction. Repeat on the other foot. **Photos M-N**

This exercise strengthens the metatarsals and limbers the ankles.

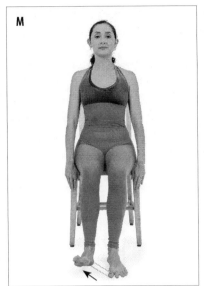
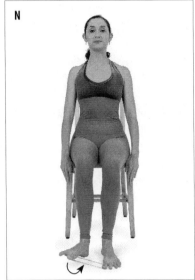

VARIATION #4:

Sitting, with the rubber band on your big toes, position one heel on the floor in line with your midline, keeping the toes and ball of that foot above the floor. Next, bend your other leg and bring it toward your chest. You can put your hands behind your thigh or on your shin. The rubber band will be perpendicular to the floor.

Keep the rubber band taut with your top foot as you pull the toes of your bottom foot down toward the floor. Perform 3 times on each foot. **Photos O-P**

This exercise strengthens the bottom of the foot. It is similar to the Towel Footwork.

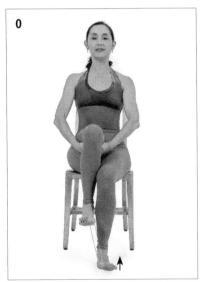
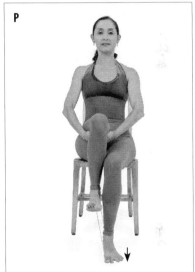

VARIATION #5:

Sitting, with the rubber band on your big toes, position one foot flat on the floor, in line with your midline. Next, bend the other leg and bring it toward your chest. You can place your hands behind your thigh or on your shin. The rubber band will be perpendicular to the floor.

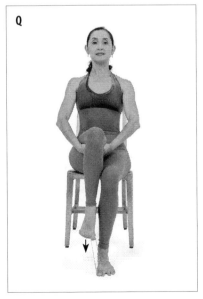
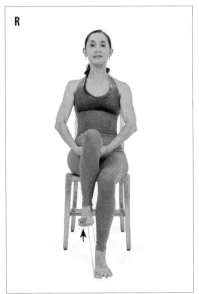

Keep your bottom foot on the floor as you pull the toes of your raised foot toward the ceiling. Flex your top foot 3 times and repeat on the other foot. **Photos Q-R on page 17.**

This exercise strengthens the top of the foot and the front of the shin.

Why It's Beneficial
The Rubber Band Exercises mimic the exercises performed with the Toe Corrector apparatus, also known as the Magic Square for the toes. The slight resistance from the rubber band is the key. These exercises help you connect to your powerhouse muscles as you open the metatarsals, work the transverse arches, and develop mobility in the toes and ankles. These exercises also strengthen the seat and outer thighs. They are appropriate for people with healthy feet and for people who have developed bunions and hammertoes.

Tips
Try to think about your toes when you are outside the Pilates studio. Stretch the tips of your socks before putting socks on and make sure that the box of your closed toed shoes gives you enough room to spread your toes.

Eventually
Unlike the first five Rubber Band Exercises, the following exercise with the rubber band doesn't use the floor to provide support. It should be introduced last in the series.

VARIATION #6:
To start, sit on the mat with your legs extended in front of you, parallel and apart. Students with stiff backs and/or tight hamstrings can bend the knees slightly. Your legs are parallel and apart, and your knees are soft as your heels rest on the floor.

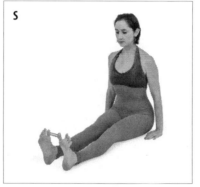 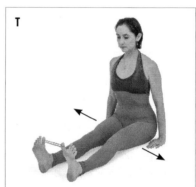

Lengthen your spine as you squeeze your seat, pull your bellybutton in and up, and use your inner thighs to energetically hug the midline of your body. To get a good starting position, with flexed feet and toes straight up, imagine that your feet are pieces of toast in the slots of a toaster oven. This next step is very important: put a little tension on the rubber band by squeezing your seat in, and pressing your outer thigh muscles away from each other. **Photos S-T**

With your feet parallel and apart and your rubber band staying taut, push the balls of your feet forward, extending your ankles, then extend your toes toward the floor. To reverse, pull your toes back, followed by the balls of your feet as you push out through your heels. Perform up to 3 sets with the feet moving in unison. **Photos U-W**

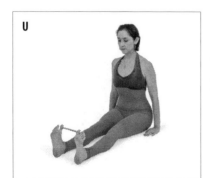 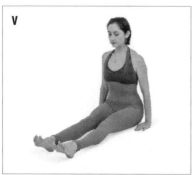 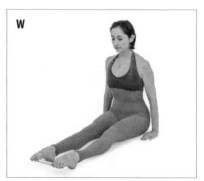

After moving the ankles and toes forward and back in unison, you can alternate, flexing one foot while pointing your other foot. Perform up to 3 sets with the feet alternating. **Photo X**

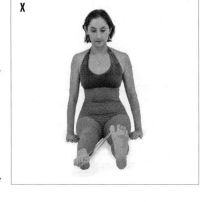

This exercise works the whole lower portion of the body: toes, feet, ankles, calves, outer thighs, and seat. It is good for those who need to work on the articulation of the feet.

FOOTWORK STANDING
Getting Started
Stand in the best position for your body: feet together, parallel and apart, or Pilates stance. With your powerhouse activated, maintain straight legs as you rise up on your toes, and straight legs as you lower your heels with control. Squeeze your seat as you lift your feet and lift your bellybutton higher as you lower your heels to the floor.

When you are able to rise up and down on your toes while keeping your weight in the center of the balls of the feet, over the second toes, you can move on to the full Footwork Standing sequence. There are four parts to the Standing Footwork exercise. First, with your powerhouse activated and your feet in the ideal stance for your body, lift your heels and rise onto your toes with straight legs **(Photo Y)**. In the second phase, keep your heels lifted and bend your knees **(Photo Z)**. In the third phase, keep your knees bent

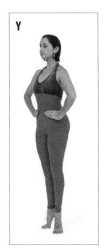 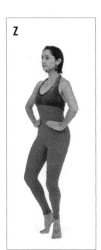 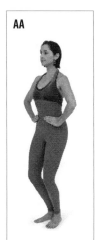 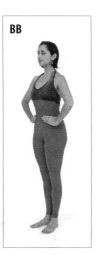

and press your heels into the floor **(Photo AA)**. Finally, keep your feet on the floor and press down through your feet as you straighten your legs **(Photo BB)**. Perform 2-3 times and reverse.

Why It's Beneficial
The Footwork Standing develops balance, strengthens the ankles, and stretches the calves and Achilles tendons. The stretch is accentuated with the use of a thick book or padded 2x4 under the balls of your feet. If you do not find the connection between engaging your powerhouse and lifting your heels, you will feel as if you are walking on stilts. As you connect your powerhouse to the movement in your feet, you will have more control in your ankles and improved balance.

Tips
If you have very flexible feet, be sure that you only lift your heels ½ to ¾ of your full capacity. This will stop the ankles at the point at which they need to work most. When performing the Footwork Standing in a Pilates stance, the heels will stay glued together throughout the duration of the exercise, which provides more balance support. If the heels separate in the Pilates stance variation of the Standing Footwork, the heels have been lifted too high.

Eventually
After learning the Footwork sequence on the floor, you can perform the same sequence with the toes and balls

of the feet on a thick book. Hold the back of a chair for support. Eventually you will perform this exercise with your arms long by your sides. When you no longer need to hold something for balance, you will quickly learn to adjust your posture and range of movement in order to maintain your balance control. **Photos CC-FF**

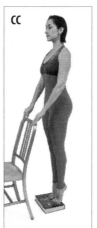 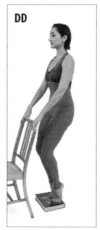 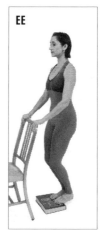 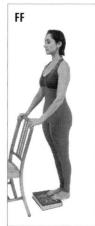

PRESSURE POINTS

Why It's Beneficial
Stimulating pressure points on the bottom of the feet is supposed to promote health throughout the body. In these exercises, a tennis ball takes the place of the Foot Corrector apparatus.

PRESSURE POINTS: TOES

Getting Started
Position a tennis ball on the floor in front of you, about a leg's distance away. Hold the seatback of a chair to improve your balance. Keep your heel on the floor as you spread your toes and wrap them around the tennis ball. Initiating the movement from your seat muscles, press down through the ball of your foot *without* shifting your weight forward. Your ankle will stretch forward slightly, but your heel should remain on the floor. Make sure that you lift up through your powerhouse as you press forward through the ball of your foot. Press into the ball and hold for three counts. Perform 3 times on each foot. **Photo GG**

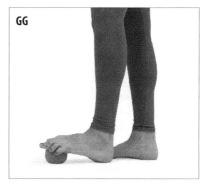

Tips
Standing farther away from the tennis ball with the heel down on the floor makes this exercise extra challenging. Direct your focus to lifting your powerhouse so that you will not resort to shifting your bodyweight forward.

Eventually
Perform the same sequence without holding the seatback of a chair for support. Visualize growing an extra inch through your waistline every time you press into the ball.

PRESSURE POINTS: ARCHES

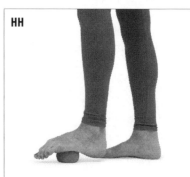

Getting Started
Put a tennis ball on the floor in front of you and place your arch on the ball. Your working leg is slightly bent. Hold the seatback of a chair to improve your balance. *Without* shifting your weight forward, press down through the arch of your foot as you engage your powerhouse muscles. Press into the ball and hold for three counts. Perform 3 times on each foot. **Photo HH**

Note
The arch can be a sensitive spot for some people. Flat feet, high arches, excessive pronation, etc. play a roll in this sensitivity.

Make sure that you spread your toes apart before wrapping your foot around the ball on each repetition. Imagine that your foot is wrapped around the ball like the talons of a bird wrapped around a perch.

Eventually
While holding onto something for balance is okay, placing the arms genie-style with the forearms stacked and elbows lifted is the ideal choice for this exercise.

PRESSURE POINTS: HEELS

Getting Started
Put a tennis ball on the floor in front of you. Hold the seatback of a chair to improve your balance. With your toes *on the floor* in front of the ball, press your heel down into the tennis ball as you engage your seat muscles and pull your bellybutton in and up. Press into the ball and hold for three counts. Perform 3 times on each foot. **Photo II**

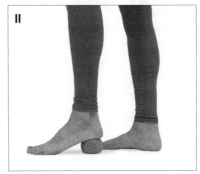

Tips
Most students are able to feel the seat muscles activate as they press down through the heel. Establishing the heel-seat connection will make jumping more powerful and will take pressure off the knees in activities such as climbing stairs and standing up from seated positions.

Eventually
Perform the same sequence without holding the seatback of a chair for support. Make sure that you don't shift your weight forward to press into the ball. Keep your weight on your supporting leg and activate your seat muscles to press through your heel.

FOOT MASSAGE

Why It's Beneficial
Rolling the bottom of the foot over a tennis ball or rolling pin provides a foot massage similar to the one on the Foot Corrector, without the risk of getting pinched by the Foot Corrector pegs. It stimulates the pressure points on the bottom of the feet.

Getting Started
Place a tennis ball or a rolling pin on the floor in front of you. Since you will be shifting your weight forward, it is a good idea to hold the seatback of a chair for balance. As you slide your foot forward over the pin or ball, let your toes drip off the front and slide along the floor as your heel presses into the pin or ball. As you repeat the foot massage with your heel sliding back over the pin or ball in the opposite direction, imagine that you are scraping mud off the bottom of your shoe. Perform 3-5 sets of the forward and backward motion on each foot. **Photo JJ**

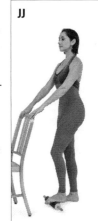

Tips
No matter what part of the foot is pressing into the rolling pin, keep the same amount of pressure on it.

Eventually
Perform the same sequence without holding the seatback of a chair for support.

PRE-PILATES FOR THE KNEES

INTRODUCTION

After I retired from my career as a professional ballet dancer, I took up flamenco dancing as a pastime. Despite my ballet background, flamenco dancing was harder than I had anticipated. I developed severe knee pain as a result of my inability to stamp my feet without tensing my legs. It hurt to walk down stairs and to stand up from a seated position. I reached the point at which the lightest spring setting on the Reformer Footwork exercise was too much resistance. Before going to a doctor, I decided to do the Pre-Pilates Leg Raises and TV Exercises. With consistent practice of the Pre-Pilates knee exercises twice a day and improved technique in my Flamenco dancing, my knee pain disappeared completely in a matter of weeks. Despite being a bit monotonous to perform, the Pre-Pilates knee exercises are highly effective, safe, and easy to practice on your own.

LEG RAISES

Getting Started

Lie on your back and rest your feet on the mat with your legs bent at a ninety-degree angle. Extend one leg on the mat in parallel and focus on buttoning your bellybutton to the mat, squeezing your seat and using your inner thighs to hug your midline. With your powerhouse muscles activated, lift your extended leg to the level of your bent knee. The supporting leg is bent at a ninety-degree angle and the extended leg should be at a forty-five degree angle above the mat.

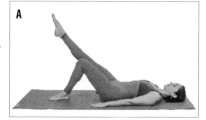 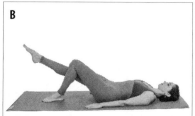

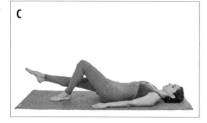 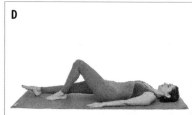

You can let your working leg touch the inside of the knee of your supporting leg. Hold the leg at knee height from three counts to ten counts. Then lower the working leg to the calf of your bent leg for another three to ten counts. Next, lower your working leg to the ankle of your bent leg for three to ten counts. <u>Before lifting the working leg back to forty-five degrees, be sure to rest your leg on the mat for a moment.</u> **Photos A-D**

Perform 3 sets of Leg Raises, each set consists of holding the leg at the knee, calf, and ankle, then resting the leg on the mat. Repeat the 3 sets on the other leg. If one of the knees is delicate, perform the Leg Raises with the weak leg first, then on the stronger side, and finish with another 3 sets of Leg Raises on the weak side.

To give this exercise some variety, do the Leg Raises in the reverse order, starting from the ankle, working up to the knee, and resting the leg on the mat after each set.

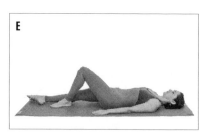

The working leg can also be held in Pilates stance for this exercise. This variation will shift the focus from strengthening the top of the thigh, the quadriceps muscle, to strengthening the inside of the working knee. **Photo E**

Why It's Beneficial

The Leg Raises strengthen the muscles in the legs and improve muscle strength around the knees. "Simply walking up or down stairs can place as much as six-hundred pounds of pressure on the patella" (Biel 245). The

Leg Raises are not the most interesting exercises in the Pilates Method, but they are a safe and highly effective way of strengthening the quadriceps and the area around the knees.

Tips
Instead of relying on ankle weights for resistance, focus on keeping the back of the knee soft while holding the leg in the air. Adding weight to the working leg only makes it tempting to hyperextend the knee. Keeping tension out of the knee joint gives the muscles the chance to do the work.

Eventually
For more challenge, perform the Leg Raises with the working leg near, but not touching the supporting leg.

TV EXERCISES

Getting Started
Sit on the front edge of a chair with your feet parallel and apart on the floor. Your legs are bent at ninety degrees and your arms are long by your sides or crossed with your forearms overlapped and your elbows lifted. Keeping your powerhouse engaged, hips and shoulders even, and without allowing your torso to lean back, keep your knee bent and lift your knee and foot away from the floor for three to ten counts. **Photo F**

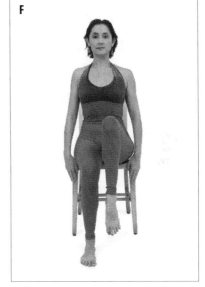

F

Perform 3 times on one side and 3 times on the other leg. If one knee is weaker, start with 3 knee lifts on the weaker side, followed by 3 lifts on the stronger side, and add 3 more lifts on the weaker side.

Why It's Beneficial
Romana nicknamed these knee lifts "TV Exercises" because she gave them as homework that could be done almost anywhere, even while sitting and watching television. The TV Exercises strengthen the quadriceps and the area around the knees. They require powerhouse strength and body awareness because there is no support for the back, and because it is challenging to keep the evenness in the frame of the body as one leg lifts. The frame of the body is formed my connecting the dots from shoulder to shoulder, hip to hip, and from each shoulder to its respective hip.

Tips
Use opposing lines of energy as you lift your bent knee. As you push your supporting foot down into the floor, your working knee will lift and so will your powerhouse.

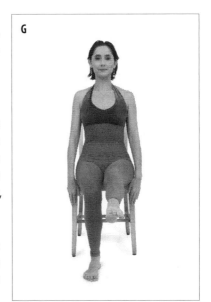

G

Eventually
For an added challenge you can perform the Pre-Pilates Leg Raises while seated. Extend one leg forward on the floor, then lift it for three to ten counts. The leg may be parallel, or rotated in Pilates stance. The goal is to lift the leg without letting the upper body lean back. Perform 3 leg lifts on the first side, repeat on the second side, or do weak side, strong side, weak side. **Photo G**

For a bigger challenge, lift one bent knee and extend the leg forward. Then lower the leg to the floor and slide the foot back to starting position. The knee lift combined with the extension of the leg resembles the leg motion of riding a bicycle. Do this three times on one side, then three times on the other side. The bicycle motion may also be done in reverse. For a more difficult challenge, the legs can alternate as they perform the bicycle movement in one direction, then in the other direction.

GOING BEYOND PRE-PILATES FOR THE KNEES

SIDE LEG KICKS

Why It's Beneficial
Keep your knees healthy by balancing strengthening exercises, such as the Leg Raises and the TV Exercises, with exercises that stretch your legs. The Side Leg Kick exercise that moves from front to back will stretch the back of the thigh as the leg moves forward and the top of the thigh as the leg moves back.

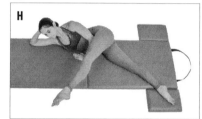

Getting Started
Lie on one side and prop your head with your bottom hand. Put your other hand on the mat in front of your waist. Your elbow, shoulder, waist and hip are in line with the back edge of the mat. Your legs form an obtuse angle with your upper body as you position your feet off the front edge of the mat.

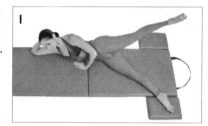

Turn your top leg out at your hip, lengthen it beyond your bottom leg, and lift it so that it is level with your working hip. Kick your leg toward your nose to the front **(Photo H)**, and kick it toward the back edge of the mat **(Photo I)**. Perform 8-10 times.

Tips
Keep your hips stacked by rotating your top leg outward in Pilates stance as it goes in front of your supporting leg, and rotating it slightly inward in parallel as it goes behind your supporting leg.

Eventually
Instead of leaving your hand on the mat by your waist, put it behind your head to challenge your balance control.

BRIDGE
Strong hamstrings are just as important as strong quadriceps for maintaining healthy knees. See the full description of the Bridge on page 26, in the section that describes Pre-Pilates for the hips. **Photo J**

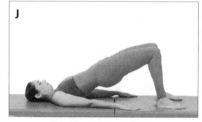

PRE-PILATES FOR THE HIPS

INTRODUCTION
I have a lot of flexibility in my hips and that is probably part of the reason that I never experienced any hip pain throughout my dancing career. It's been twenty years since the last time I danced onstage and I can no longer boast about having injury-free hip joints. I have developed tendonitis in my left hip which, when it flares up, is extremely painful. Simply lifting my leg to put pants on can cause pain when my tendonitis is aggravated. It

is the type of injury that requires a lot of patience, as resting the hip does not seem to make a difference. I do Pre-Pilates hip exercises when I experience flare-ups and I also do them to build back the strength in my hips.

TOWEL UNDER THE THIGH

Getting Started
Lie on your back and rest your feet on the mat with bent legs. Then, bring one knee toward you and hook a rolled towel underneath the thigh of your bent leg. Imagine that your thigh is resting in a hammock. Using your arms to hold the towel, gently pull the towel toward you for three seconds and then release. Perform 3 times on each leg. If necessary, start with the delicate hip, repeat on the other side, and then do an additional set on the weaker side. **Photo A**

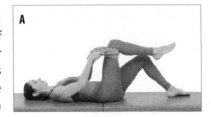

Tips
The working leg should feel like dead weight as it rests in the towel. It is the towel, powered by the arms, that moves the leg.

Eventually
When you are ready for an added stretch, you can use the towel to move the thigh in a small circular motion. Perform up to 5 small circles in one direction and then reverse. Repeat on the other leg. If necessary, start with the delicate hip, repeat on the other side, and then do an additional set on the weaker side.

Why It's Beneficial
This exercise is a modified version of the Single Leg Circles. Like the Single Leg Circles, it works the leg in the hip socket, but the use of the towel provides additional support for the leg as it moves.

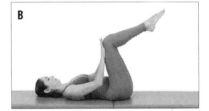

PRESSURE ON THE THIGHS

Getting Started
To strengthen the area around the hip sockets, lie on your back and bring your knees toward your chest. Next, position your hands on the tops of your thighs and push the tops of your thighs against your hands, as the hands resist the pressure for three seconds **(Photo B)**. To work the opposing line of energy, reposition your hands behind your thighs and push the backs of your thighs against your hands, as the hands resist the pressure for three seconds **(Photo C)**. Perform 3 times with the hands on the tops of the thighs and 3 times with the hands on the backs of the thighs.

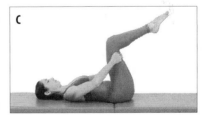

Next, place your hands on the outside of your thighs and press your outer thighs into your hands as your hands resist the pressure for three seconds **(Photo D)**. To work the opposing line of energy, reposition the palms of the hands on the inner thighs with the wrists crossed. As the inner thighs press toward the body's midline, the hands resist the pressure for three seconds **(Photo E)**.

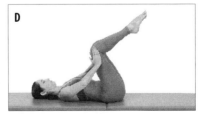

Why It's Beneficial
Using the hands to create resistance in different places on the thighs builds strength in the inner and outer thighs and hip flexors. These exercises are extremely helpful for creating stability in the hip joints.

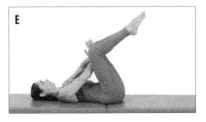

Tips
As you activate the muscles in your legs and around your hips, be sure that you maintain the integrity of your leg alignment from the hip, through the knee, to the ankle.

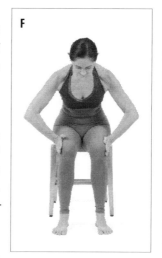 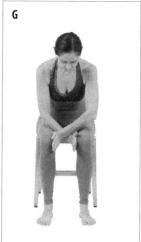

Eventually
Sit at the front edge of a chair with your feet and legs parallel and apart. Place your hands on the outside of your thighs and press your outer thighs into your hands as your hands resist the pressure for three seconds (**Photo F**). To work the opposing line of energy, reposition the palms of the hands on the inner thighs with the wrists crossed. As the inner thighs press toward the body's midline, the hands resist the pressure for three seconds (**Photo G**). Perform 3 times on the outer thighs and 3 times on the inner thighs.

Next, position your hands on the tops of your thighs and push the tops of your thighs against your hands. As your hands resist the pressure from your legs, lift your heels off the floor. To work the opposing line of energy, keep your heels raised with your toes on the floor and reposition your hands behind your thighs. As your hands resist the pressure from the backs of your thighs, lower your heels to the floor.

BRIDGE

Getting Started
Lie on your back with your legs bent at a ninety-degree angle, feet resting on the mat. Your feet and legs are parallel and hip bone width apart. Engage your powerhouse muscles, lift your pelvis, and hold the bridge shape for three counts. Perform 3-5 times. **Photo H**

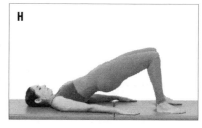

Why It's Beneficial
The Bridge stabilizes the pelvis, strengthens the seat muscles, and stretches the front of the hips. People who spend a lot of time sitting can get tight hip flexors. The Bridge is the perfect antidote to long hours spent in the seated position.

Tips
Remember to engage your seat muscles otherwise you may develop cramps in the backs of your legs to compensate for the lack of energy in the buttocks muscles.

Eventually
When you are ready, emphasize the deliberate articulation of the spine as the tailbone, low back, waist, and upper back peel off the mat to make the bridge shape. After holding the bridge shape for three seconds, "melt" your sternum, ribs, waist, and hips into the mat. Perform 3-5 times.

GOING BEYOND
PRE-PILATES FOR THE HIPS

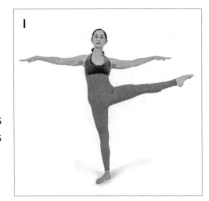

ONE LEG BALANCE

The One Leg Balance comes from Joe's archival standing exercises. It works the hip as one leg extends front, side, or back. See pages 95-96 in the Joe's Archival Routine chapter for details. **Photo I**

SINGLE LEG CIRCLES

When you are ready to progress from the Towel Under the Thigh exercise, do the Single Leg Circles to work the leg in the hip socket while strengthening the sides of the torso. See pages 76-77 in the Basic Matwork with a Towel chapter for details on the Single Leg Circles. **Photo J**

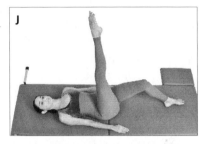

PRE-PILATES FOR THE BACK

INTRODUCTION

About fifteen years ago I sprained my back. I didn't do anything extreme to bring on my back injury. I was at a restaurant watching a show in a very uncomfortable seat. After spending the evening fidgeting in my chair I went to bed later that same night and woke up with intense back pain. Everyday tasks like putting groceries in the refrigerator were almost impossible. I knew that I needed to move to improve the circulation in and around my injury so I did the Pre-Pilates back exercises and eventually moved up to the Basic Matwork. My delicate back forced me to work from my abdominal muscles as opposed to relying on momentum from my limbs. I don't think I have ever worked as deeply in my powerhouse as I did when I sprained my back. Unfortunately, this was not my only experience with back pain.

I was diagnosed with osteopenia in my spine in my early twenties. The intensity of my exercise routine as a professional dancer had caused me to have amenorrhea for five years, which triggered estrogen deficiency and poor calcium absorption. I was able to reverse the osteopenia in my thirties, with the help of Pilates and the absence of a rigorous dance schedule. Now in my forties, the osteopenia has returned. One of the principal reasons I do Pilates is to avoid back pain. No matter how my back feels, if I can walk into the Pilates studio, I know that I can find Pilates exercises that will make me feel better.

For students with back pain, the Pre-Pilates exercises for the back are safe and effective because they are performed with back support. While the traditional Pilates moves are very good for limbering the spine and strengthening back muscles, movements that incorporate forward flexion, back extension, side bends, and twists are not always appropriate for students who have back problems and/or who lack significant Pilates experience. Additionally, Pre-Pilates exercises for the back can be educational. They help students recognize that the powerhouse muscles must be engaged in order to maintain the integrity of the back placement as the limbs move through space. Whether your back is delicate or healthy, the Pre-Pilates exercises for the back will make a good addition to your regular Pilates routine at home.

HUG KNEE(S) TO CHEST
Getting Started
Lie on your back with your legs bent and feet resting on the mat. Sink your bellybutton into the mat as you draw

one knee to your chest. Stack your hands, no interlaced fingers, on your shin or ankle as you gently pull your thigh to your chest. **Photo A**

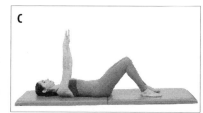

Why It's Beneficial
Gently hugging the knee(s) to the chest stretches the low back and often relieves low back pain.

Tips
Students with delicate knees can hold the back of the thigh to reduce pressure on the knee as the thigh comes to the chest. The thigh is hugged with gentle pressure and the hips remain anchored as the leg bends.

Eventually
For a deeper stretch, bring both knees to the chest. To avoid back strain at the start of the stretch, bend one knee to the chest at a time. Once both knees are to the chest, pull the thighs toward you gently, or draw tiny circles with the knees to massage the back. Draw circles with the knees 3 times in each direction. To come out of the stretch without putting strain on the back, rest one foot on the floor before lowering the other foot. **Photo B**

MOVING THE LIMBS AWAY FROM THE CENTER

Getting Started
Lie on your back with your arms stretched toward the ceiling and your legs bent at ninety degrees, feet resting on the mat **(Photo C)**. Take a deep breath to prepare for the movement and extend one arm back, away from your bellybutton, as you breathe out **(Photo D)**. The arm can reach beside the ear, but should not go all the way to the mat. To keep tension out of your shoulder, remember to slide your shoulder blade down into your back as the arm reaches toward the ear. To complete the movement, return your arm to the starting position as you breathe in. Perform 1-2 times on each arm and then rest the arms on the mat.

A version of this exercise is also done with the legs. Keeping the back flat on the mat, position your feet and legs hip bone width apart and legs bent **(Photo E)**. After a deep breath, exhale as you slide one foot forward on the mat **(Photo F)**. *Observe* what happens to your back as you move your foot and leg away from your center, and *anticipate* when to stop moving your leg. Not everyone will be able to stretch the leg completely. Breathe in as the knee returns to starting position. Perform 1-2 times on each leg.

Why It's Beneficial
This exercise teaches you the importance of pulling deeper into your powerhouse muscles as you move your limbs away from the center of your body. It coordinates the breath with the movement of the limbs and helps center the mind as well as the body.

Tips
The Footwork Series at the beginning of the Reformer workout helps center the body alignment and mental focus. When performing the Matwork, you can do the Moving the Limbs Away From the Center exercise before the Hundred to help center your body alignment and mental focus.

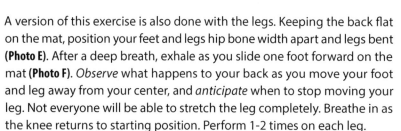
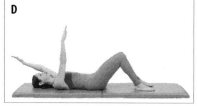
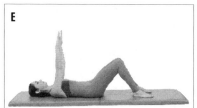
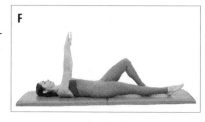

Eventually

When you are ready, you can practice moving one arm back toward your ear as one foot slides forward on the mat. Beginning in home position with the arms perpendicular to the mat and the legs bent at ninety degrees, take a deep breath to prepare, and breathe out while extending one arm back and one leg forward. To challenge the coordination, move your right arm back as your left foot slides forward. Breathe in to return to home position and repeat with the left arm and right foot sliding away from each other. Perform 2 sets, breathing out as the limbs extend away from the powerhouse and breathing in to return to home position. **Photos G-H**

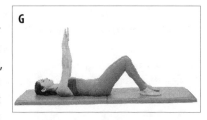

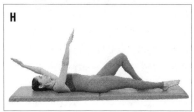

LEG RAISES

Although the Leg Raises are traditionally considered a Pre-Pilates exercise for the knees, the Leg Raises can just as easily be performed with attention to the back placement. You learn that it is harder to button your bellybutton to the mat as your working leg gets closer to the mat. See page 22 in the Pre-Pilates for the Knees section of this chapter for more details. **Photo I**

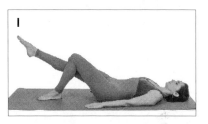

GOING BEYOND PRE-PILATES FOR THE BACK

HAMSTRING STRETCH

Tight hamstrings can cause discomfort in the back. Do Hamstring Stretches with the back supported on the mat to help maintain flexibility in the backs of the legs. Put a towel on the sole of your foot and gently pull the ends of the towel to deepen the stretch. See pages 75-76 in the Basic Matwork with a Towel chapter for details on the Hamstring Stretches that precede the Single Leg Circles. **Photo J**

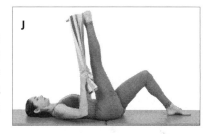

Eventually

As you gain flexibility, you can replace the towel with the Magic Circle. Place the inside cushion of the Magic Circle over the ball of your foot. Stretch your leg toward the ceiling while pulling gently on the circle. In time, you can move your supporting foot farther away from your seat, eventually stretching your bottom leg out on the mat while stretching your top leg. Perform 1-3 times on each leg, for no more than three seconds at a time. **Photo K**

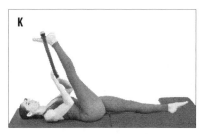

MAGIC CIRCLE ARMS

Getting Started

Lie on your back with your legs stretched on the mat. Hold the Magic Circle between the palms of your hands, fingertips extended. Extend your arms toward the ceiling at an angle so that the circle is just above your waistline. Keeping your arms long and your elbows soft, pull your bellybutton in as you press into the circle for three counts. Perform 3-5 times. **Photo L**

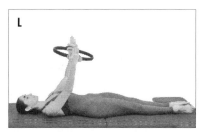

Why It's Beneficial

This exercise strengthens the arms and helps you find the connection between your back muscles and your arms. It teaches you that engaging the abdominal muscles allows for more powerful movement in the arms in addition to helping with the correct back placement on the mat.

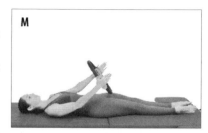

Eventually

For an extra challenge, take the Magic Circle farther away from your power-house. First, reach toward your toes, with the circle above your thighs, and press into the circle for three counts (**Photo M**). Perform 3-5 times. Next, lift the circle back toward your ears, keeping your arms within your peripheral vision. With long arms, soft elbows, and powerhouse muscles activated, press into the circle and hold the pressure for three seconds. When your arms are near your ears, you have to work extra hard to keep your ribcage closed and your back anchored (**Photo N**). Perform 3-5 times.

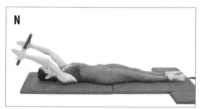

MAGIC CIRCLE LEGS

Getting Started

Lie on your back with your legs bent at a ninety-degree angle, feet parallel and hip bone width apart on the mat. Place the Magic Circle between your inner thighs, just above your knees. With your powerhouse engaged, use your inner thighs to squeeze the circle. Hold the pressure on the circle for three seconds before releasing it. Perform 3-5 times. **Photo O**

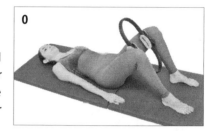

Eventually

For an extra challenge, place the Magic Circle perpendicular to the mat, a leg's distance away from you with your ankles inside the circle to hold it in place. Lie on your back with your legs stretched and keep one ankle inside the circle, resting over the bottom cushion, and put your other ankle outside the circle, over the top cushion. With your legs extended and knees soft, pull your bellybutton in and squeeze your seat as you gently press your top leg down on the circle for three counts. Perform 3 times on each leg. **Photos P-Q**

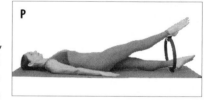

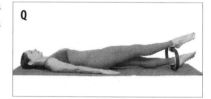

Tips

For the Getting Started variation, make sure that you are using your inner thighs, not your knees, to move the circle. To check for evenness in the body in the Eventually variation, imagine that you have the Short Pole across your waistline. Don't let it wobble as you move the Magic Circle.

Why It's Beneficial

The Getting Started variation strengthens the seat and inner thigh muscles. The Eventually variation strengthens the backs of the legs and can be used to even out muscle imbalances in the body. The mat provides back support in both variations.

PRE-PILATES FOR BALANCE

INTRODUCTION

As a dancer, my flexibility was greater than my strength and control. I really had to resist sinking into my joints as I attempted to balance on one leg. Because poor balance affects one's gait, I used to hyperextend my knees and sink into my hips as I walked with my feet too far apart, and with my toes pointing outward like a duck's webs. One day, as I was walking along the beach, I heard a group of children giggling. Curious, I looked back to see what they were doing. I was embarrassed when I realized that they were stepping in my overly turned out footprints in the sand!

Years later, at the start of my training to become a certified Pilates teacher, the very first task I received was to walk across the room. The master teacher who taught the intensive seminar at the start of my apprenticeship had a true talent for reproducing a person's gait with uncanny accuracy. After each newbie walked across the room, she replicated their gait. I found it quite entertaining until I watched her mimic my gait. It looked so exaggerated and inelegant as she sank into her hips and kept her feet too far apart as she walked! I was reminded of that day on the beach when the children were giggling as they stepped in my footprints. I thought that I had corrected my gait, but based on her accurate imitation of everyone else in the studio, I knew that her imitation of my gait was spot on.

Many of the exercises in this section have taught me to be more mindful of my gait. They teach you to walk with correct posture, keeping the weight forward on the feet while aligning the knees over the toes. They also emphasize how to shift the body weight efficiently. Additionally, the exercises in this section focus on the muscles necessary for improving balance control when standing on one leg.

People often think that balancing on one leg only requires a strong ankle and strong muscles in the foot, but people who attempt to balance using only these muscles have little success. Pilates training teaches students to shift their focus from their extremities into their center. They learn to work from above the knee into the powerhouse, lifting through the thigh, hip, and waistline, instead of focusing on the leg from the knee down.

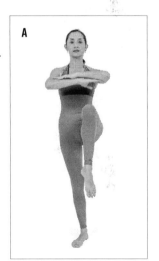

MARCHING
Getting Started
Stand tall with your feet close together, forearms stacked and elbows lifted. Alternate lifting one knee at a time toward your chest. Your foot barely touches the floor before your other foot comes up. It is tempting to sacrifice the lift in the body in order to lift the knee higher. Think of lifting your torso higher as your knee comes toward your chest. Perform up to 20 knee lifts. **Photo A**

To stretch the backs of the legs while working the balance on one leg, brush your foot along the floor in front of you and lift your leg straight to the front as high as you can manage without disrupting the evenness in your hips and shoulders. Alternate kicking one leg at a time to the front. Perform up to 20 kicks. **Photo B**

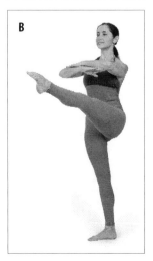

Why It's Beneficial
The Marching exercise develops balance control and strengthens the supporting hip.

Tips
Be sure that the accent is on the upbeat with the knee in the air. A good way to keep the accent on the upbeat is to imagine that the floor is scorching hot.

Eventually
For an added challenge, the Marching exercise can be done with the knee lifting to the side. It is much harder to maintain the integrity of the box, shoulder to shoulder,

and hip to hip evenness, when lifting the leg to the side. Stand with your arms extended to the side and pay attention to the placement of your rib cage as you perform this variation of the Marching exercise. **Photo C**

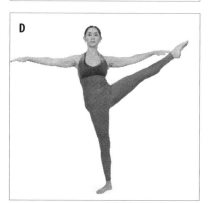

To deepen the stretch in your inner thighs while working your balance on one leg, brush your foot along the floor to your side and lift your leg straight out to the side. Alternate kicking one leg at a time to the side. Perform up to 20 kicks. **Photo D**

GLIDING STEP
Getting Started

With your powerhouse lifted and your hips and shoulders even, extend your arms forward as you skim the ball of one foot forward on the floor. Next, lift the heel of your back foot off the floor as you transfer your weight onto the front foot, bringing the heel of your front foot onto the floor. The back leg will bend and the ball of that foot will pass the front foot to take the next step. Make sure that the back heel lifts before the front heel touches the floor. The balls of the feet will never leave the floor as you perform the Gliding Step. You alternate steps as you glide across the room, pressing through the ball of your foot first, and finishing with your heel as you transfer your weight onto the front leg. **Photos E-H**

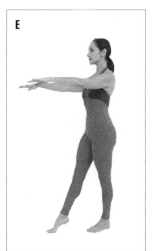
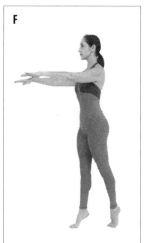
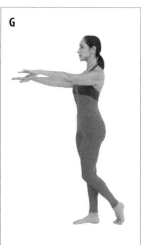
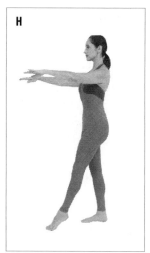

Why It's Beneficial

Toe-to-heel walking as an exercise recruits different muscles in the legs than regular heel-to-toe walking does, and it helps develop coordination and increased muscle control. The Gliding Step teaches you to transfer your body weight from toe to heel and serves as a good introductory exercise to the Goose Step. It teaches the transition of body weight between the feet without the added distraction of balancing on one leg.

Tips

Joe Pilates taught the Gliding Step to students who wore his posture apparatus. The posture apparatus was worn on the crown of the head and had two sand bags dangling from strings, one on each side of the body (Gallagher and Kryzanowska 168-169). In an interview with *Collier's, The National Weekly*, Joe described how one could build this apparatus, "Get a broomstick, suspend a sandbag holding about three pounds of sand by a cord from each end, and tie it across a deck tennis ring… Slowly, slowly stretch the left foot forward as far as you can; when the toe touches, shift the weight slowly to the left foot… the exercise done ten minutes daily will produce such a consciousness of queenly carriage that soon you'll walk beautifully without your pole" (Carr 30). You can balance a beanbag or a book on the top of your head as you perform the Gliding Step to mimic the feeling of using Joe's posture apparatus.

Eventually
For an added challenge, perform the Gliding Step in reverse. The reverse Gliding Step will resemble the Moonwalk dance move. With your powerhouse lifted and your hips and shoulders even, extend your arms forward as you skim the ball of one foot behind you on the floor. Next, lift your front heel off the floor as you transfer your weight onto the back foot, bringing the heel of your back foot to the floor. The front leg will bend and the ball of that foot will pass the back foot to take the next step. Continue to alternate steps as you glide across the room, pressing through the ball of your foot first and finishing with your heel as you transfer your weight onto the back leg.

GOOSE STEP
Getting Started
Stand upright with your powerhouse lifted and your arms extended forward at shoulder level, palms facing the floor. Begin by lifting one knee to nearly hip level. The lower half of your raised leg should be free of tension. Next, extend the lower half of your raised leg, lift your supporting heel, and prepare to step forward onto the ball of your front foot. As you transfer your weight, your front heel touches the floor and your other knee lifts in front of you. Make sure that you have your balance on one leg before you take the next step. Emphasize a small hold when balancing on one leg. Continue stepping forward in this pattern. By stepping onto the ball of your foot first and then your heel, instead of heel, ball, toes, you will develop more control and strength in your ankles and hips. This exercise should be performed with control, not speed. **Photos I-L**

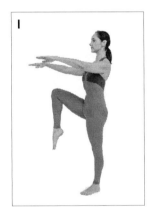 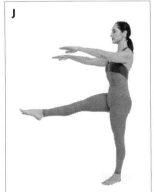 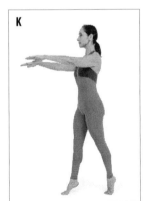 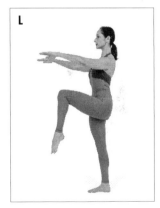

Why It's Beneficial
The Pilates version of the Goose Step is a hybrid of the military goose step typically performed with stiff legs and the high step performed with a bent knee. The Pilates Goose Step should be introduced after learning the Gliding Step and the Marching exercise. It develops coordination, body control, and balance.

The Goose Step helps you develop the muscles necessary for a healthy gait. It teaches you the importance of maintaining alignment along the hip, knee, and toes. It teaches you to keep your body weight forward as you walk, and it teaches you to lift out of your hips as you take steps.

Tips
If your supporting foot swivels on the floor when you lift your knee, you are probably sinking into your supporting hip. Remember to activate your seat muscles as you lift your torso up and press your supporting foot down into

the ground. Soon you will notice that using two opposing lines of energy gives you more stability.

Eventually
For an extra challenge, practice the Goose Step walking backward. Lift up and out of your hips as you lift your knee in front of you. After finding your balance on one leg, extend your raised leg behind you and place the ball of your back foot on the floor. As you transfer your weight onto the back leg, your heel touches the floor and your front knee lifts in front of you. Each time you transfer your weight onto the back leg, think of growing taller as you roll through the ball and heel of your supporting foot. This is very challenging!

GOING BEYOND PRE-PILATES FOR BALANCE

PILATES LUNGES

Getting Started
Stand in Pilates stance and move one heel forward so that it touches the inside of the arch of your other foot. Hold a rolling pin in your hands and extend your arms forward to help you feel shoulder evenness. Engage your powerhouse and extend your front foot forward, just beyond your leg's length. To go into the forward lunge, lower your front foot to the floor as you bend your front leg. Make sure that the middle of your front knee lines up with your second toe. Your weight should be forward on the bent leg and very light on your back foot, the straight leg. **Photo M**

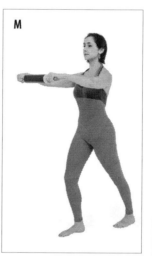
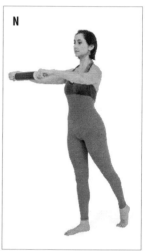

As you engage the muscles around the hip of your front leg, shift your weight forward even more as your back heel lifts off the floor **(Photo N)**. Toes stay on the floor. As you shift your weight forward, your front leg straightens. Try lifting your back heel up and putting it down without letting your weight rock back into your back leg.

Once you are comfortable keeping minimal weight in your back leg as you move your back heel up and down, you can balance on one leg, with your front leg straightening to become your supporting leg as your back knee moves and lifts in front of you **(Photo O)**. After balancing on one leg, go back into the lunge by lowering your raised leg to the floor behind you as your front leg bends **(Photos P-Q)**. <u>Make sure that you do not shift your weight onto your back foot as your foot goes to the floor while you are in the lunge position.</u> Perform 3 times on each side.

Why It's Beneficial
Like the Goose Step, the Pilates Lunges teach you to lift up and out of your hips with your weight forward on the balls of your feet. The Pilates Lunges teach you how to maintain your balance while standing on one foot. In addition to working the balance and strengthening the supporting hip, the forward lunge position strengthens the muscles in the lunging leg.

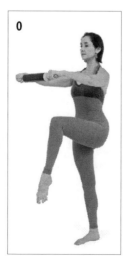
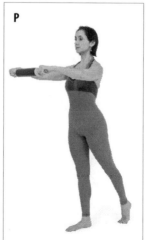
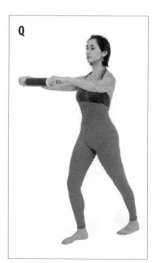

Tips

Before learning Pilates Lunges, you should be proficient in the Marching exercise. As you balance on one leg, imagine that you are still standing on two legs. This will help you maintain evenness in your hips. Once you have mastered your balance on each foot, you can practice balancing on one leg at a time, with your eyes closed for an added challenge.

Eventually

For an extra challenge you can go beyond lifting your back knee in front of you and extend your working leg forward with control. Be sure that your supporting leg stays stretched as the working leg extends forward. After demonstrating good balance control, take your front leg back into the bent knee shape and finish with your working leg reaching to the floor behind you to go back into the starting lunge position.

GOING UP FRONT WITH A LOW STOOL

Getting Started

Stand on the floor behind a low stool, and focus on maintaining evenness through the frame of your body by connecting the dots from hip to hip, shoulder to shoulder, and from each shoulder to its respective hip. With your powerhouse muscles activated, place one foot on the low stool. The leg is bent. The foot on the low stool can be positioned parallel or in Pilates stance. As you push your foot down into the low stool you will simultaneously lengthen your spine and pull up through your seat, hip, stomach, and along the sides of your waist. Remember to activate your seat muscles to give you power as you step up onto the low stool. As you straighten your front leg, your back foot leaves the floor. **Photos R-T**

With practice, you can take your back knee forward **(Photo U)**. Be sure that you do not shift your weight back onto your heel as your foot returns to the floor. Perform 3 times on each leg.

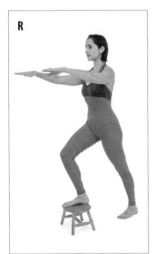 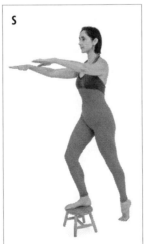 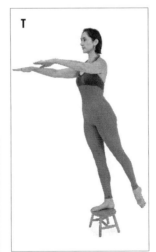 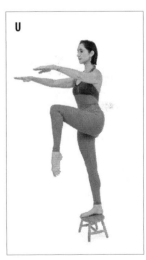

Why It's Beneficial

The Going Up Front exercise with a low stool strengthens the hip of the leg that is on top of the low stool. It mimics the Going Up Front exercise on the Electric Chair and the Front Balance Control exercise on the Wunda Chair. Because it resembles climbing, Going Up Front with a low stool teaches you to use your muscles instead of relying on your joints when you perform activities such as walking up stairs and climbing hills. It is a great exercise to reinforce the heel-seat connection.

Tips

Before learning Going Up Front with a low stool, you should be proficient in the Pilates Lunges, which teach you to keep the weight on your supporting leg as your working leg moves front and back.

If you step back too far from the stool when bringing your working leg to the floor, try placing a pad on the floor in the spot where you would like to land.

Eventually

Once you develop the necessary strength to step up onto the stool on one leg with the other leg bent in front of you, extend your bent leg forward while maintaining evenness in your frame. This is a parallel *developpé* front in dance terms. Be sure that you do not sacrifice the lift through your supporting leg as you stretch your working leg forward.

Another variation that is particularly useful for young dancers is to extend the back leg straight behind the body into *arabesque* after stepping up onto the stool. Imagine that your supporting foot is made up of tree roots that spread out on the low stool. In this scenario your supporting leg will be the tall tree trunk, and your working leg will be a long tree limb.

LEG PUSH DOWN WITH A CHAIR FRAME

Getting Started

Stand your leg's length distance away from a chair with a low frame beneath the seat of the chair. Place your hands on your hips or out to your sides, and put the bottom of your foot on the frame of the chair. Keep your working leg in parallel. Your standing leg can be parallel or rotated slightly in Pilates stance. Squeeze your seat and lift your bellybutton in and up as you press your foot gently into the frame of the chair for the count of three **(Photo V)**. Repeat two more times. Next, try to lift your leg an inch or two above the frame **(Photo W)**. Be sure to keep the frame of your body as even as possible as you lift your leg. Repeat two more times. Perform 3 leg push downs and 3 leg lifts on each side.

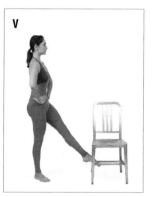 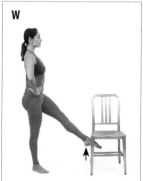

Why It's Beneficial

The Leg Push Down with a chair frame is a variation of the Leg Push Down on the Wunda Chair. It works the balance and strengthens the seat and leg muscles.

Tips

The key to this exercise is creating opposing lines of energy. As you press down through your front leg, you should feel your body lifting taller. It is also very important that you keep the backs of your knees soft so that the work stays in your muscles and does not go into your joints.

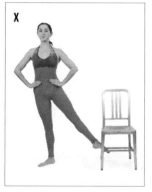 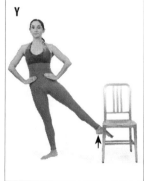

Eventually

Once you are comfortable with the Leg Push Down to the front you can do the Leg Push Down with your leg to the side. **Photos X-Y**

OTHER EXERCISES THAT GO BEYOND PRE-PILATES FOR BALANCE

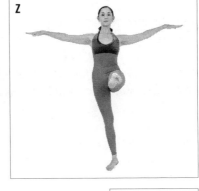

ONE LEG BALANCE
The One Leg Balance comes from Joe's archival standing exercises. It improves balance control and strengthens the supporting leg. See pages 95-96 in the Joe's Archival Routine chapter for details. **Photo Z**

TREE STANDING
This Tree exercise is a standing version of the Tree exercise performed seated on the Short Box on the Reformer. It stretches the hamstrings while working the balance control. See pages 67-68 in the Wake-Up Exercises chapter for details. **Photo AA**

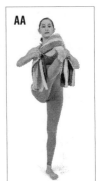

PRE-PILATES FOR THE HANDS

INTRODUCTION
I currently have four rescue dogs: a hyper Chihuahua, an overly friendly Pug/Toy Fox Terrier mix, a gentle adult Great Dane and a recently adopted Great Dane puppy. I have become quite proficient at walking my adult Great Dane and my two little dogs at the same time, but it didn't start out that way. In the early stages, every time we passed a dog on the street I went into a white-knuckled grip on their leashes for fear that the other dog might be aggressive and/or be on a retractable leash (don't get me started on those!). My frequent dog walks, plus the time I spent typing at the computer led to pain and discomfort in my finger joints. Since I depend on my hands to teach, I knew that I needed to address my pain. I turned to the Pre-Pilates exercises for the hands and began to get relief within a few weeks.

Now that I am comfortable walking the three dogs together I have another challenge, a huge Great Dane puppy! Never having adopted a puppy before, I was unprepared for the challenges of teaching such a large and energetic dog to walk on a leash. Despite working with two different trainers, she pulled me down twice. My veterinarian warned me that she has seen many clients break their wrists from such falls. She referred me to an amazing professional dog trainer who is successfully training both of us!

Exercises for the hands work not only the muscles in the hands, but also the muscles in the forearms. Here are a couple of exercises you can do anywhere:

EXERCISE #1: SPREAD THE FINGERS
To stretch the muscles in your hands, spread your fingers apart (abduction) and bring them back together (adduction) a few times. **Photos A-B**

EXERCISE #2: LIFT ONE FINGER AT A TIME
To work the fingers, practice lifting one finger at a time from a flat surface. **Photo C**

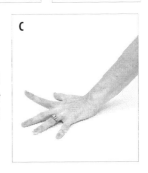

These exercises, in addition to the Pre-Pilates exercises for the hands, are a good antidote to hours spent on computers, tablets, and mobile devices. They are good for rehabilitation after healing from a fracture and/or surgery of the hand or wrist. And they are good for those who have arthritic pain in the hands.

FINGER FLICKS

Getting Started

Sit on the front edge of a chair with your feet on the floor. Legs are bent at ninety degrees. With your powerhouse activated, stretch your arms in front of you and lift them to shoulder level. With your palms facing the floor, curl your fingers into your palms, with your thumbs curled over the tips of your fingers. Flick your thumbs with the tips of your fingers as they snap out and curl back in. The movement should be brisk and crisp. Perform 3 sets of ten. **Photos D-E**

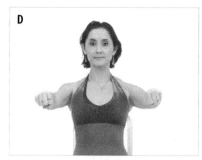

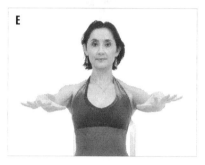

Why It's Beneficial

Part of the complexity of the human hand is due to the fact that the hands have almost a quarter of the total number of bones in the human body. Obviously, bones do not move by themselves. It takes muscles to move bones. The Finger Flicks strengthen the muscles in the hands, forearms, and underarms. Finger Flicks also stretch the fingers and the palms of the hands.

Tips

You can do the Finger Flicks to build your stamina. When I was dancing professionally, I had a Russian ballet master who gave us this exercise to help us get back into shape at the start of each ballet season. It is much harder than it appears and is very effective.

Eventually

In addition to holding your arms out at shoulder level, you can lift your arms up and down while performing the Finger Flicks. Be sure that you do not let the movement affect your posture. Finger Flicks can also be performed as the arms lift along the center of the body and circle open, the same pattern used in the Arm Circles exercise from the Wall Series. Be sure that the fingertips stay within your field of vision. Circle the arms open 2-3 times followed by 2-3 circles in the reverse direction.

WRIST CURLS

Why It's Beneficial

The Wrist Curls strengthen the hands, wrists, and forearms. In a Wrist Curl, the hand hinges at the wrist as the fingertips point to the floor and then point to the ceiling.

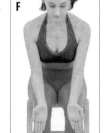

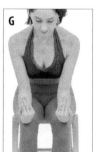

Getting Started

Sit on the front edge of a chair with your feet parallel and apart on the floor. Begin with your forearms resting on your thighs and your wrists hanging off your knees. Wrist flexion is the movement of bending the palm toward the wrist. To work your wrist flexion, turn your palms upward toward the ceiling as you alternate pointing your fingertips to the floor and curling your wrists in toward your body. **Photos F-G**

Wrist extension is the movement of raising the back of the hand. To work your wrist extension, turn your palms downward as you curl your wrists over your knees and lift your fingertips toward the ceiling. Perform 3-5 times in each direction. **Photos H-I**

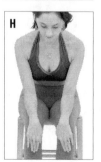

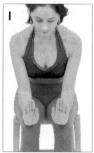

Tips

The Wrist Curls are especially useful for people who have been given a doctor's approval to start wrist strengthening exercises after the removal of a cast or after surgery.

Eventually

When you are ready for more resistance and added stretch, you can hold a one-pound weight in each hand. When doing the Wrist Curls with the palms facing upwards, try to let the weight roll toward your fingertips when the fingertips reach toward the floor. The light pressure of the weight will deepen the stretch in your wrists, fingers, and forearms.

WRIST TWIRLS/FLOREO

Getting Started

First, position your arms in a closed hug position with your palms facing you **(Photo J)**. Then, curl your wrists toward you without moving your arms, so that your fingertips point toward you **(Photo K)**. Next, your wrists roll so that your fingertips point to the floor **(Photo L)**. Continue to rotate your wrists so that your fingertips point away from your midline **(Photo M)**. To complete the Wrist Twirl, finish with your palms facing away from you and fingertips pointing toward each other **(Photo N)**. Remember to keep your elbows steady throughout the wrist movement. Reverse the movement to come back to the starting position. Perform 3-5 sets.

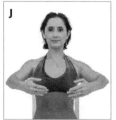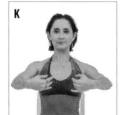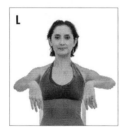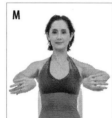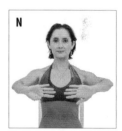

Why It's Beneficial

One of the things I remember most about Romana was how selective she was when it came to choosing restaurants. The deciding factor had very little to do with the food. For daytime dining she wanted to be al fresco. As she ate, she enjoyed watching (and critiquing) the way people walked on the sidewalk. For evening dining, she loved restaurants with live entertainment, especially dancing. Romana's love of flamenco dancing inspired the Wrist Twirls, referred to as *Floreo* in flamenco dance. They strengthen the upper arms, work the fingers, and increase mobility in the wrists.

Tips

Before you add the wrist movement, practice holding your arms in front of your body. Position your arms in a closed hug position. With your shoulder blades sliding down your back and your collar bones open, imagine that you are resting your elbows and forearms on a tabletop as you hug a large basket.

When you are ready to add the wrist movement, remember to isolate the elbows from the wrist movement. In this exercise, the arms can be thought of as stems and the hands as flowers. Without strong stems, the flowers will look like they are wilting.

Eventually

In flamenco dancing, the women and men perform the *Floreo* differently. For men, the finger movement is minimal and therefore a little easier. The four fingers of each hand remain close to one another as the wrists turn. For women, the middle fingers initiate the movement in the wrists. You can do the female version of the *Floreo* for an added challenge. To do that version of the *Floreo*, imagine that you delicately catch a butterfly between the tip of your thumb and middle finger at the start, then, after completing the wrist circle you separate your thumb and middle finger to release the butterfly. In time you can lead with the middle fingers without actually bringing the tips of the middle fingers and thumbs together. **Photo O**

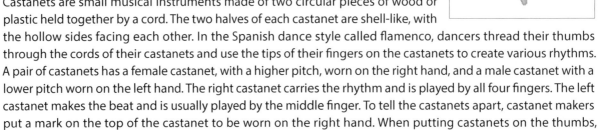

CASTANETS

What Are Castanets?

Castanets are small musical instruments made of two circular pieces of wood or plastic held together by a cord. The two halves of each castanet are shell-like, with the hollow sides facing each other. In the Spanish dance style called flamenco, dancers thread their thumbs through the cords of their castanets and use the tips of their fingers on the castanets to create various rhythms. A pair of castanets has a female castanet, with a higher pitch, worn on the right hand, and a male castanet with a lower pitch worn on the left hand. The right castanet carries the rhythm and is played by all four fingers. The left castanet makes the beat and is usually played by the middle finger. To tell the castanets apart, castanet makers put a mark on the top of the castanet to be worn on the right hand. When putting castanets on the thumbs, the side of the cord with the knot slides over the thumb first. The knot on the cord can slide to adjust tightness.

Getting Started

This exercise can be performed seated or standing, with the powerhouse muscles active. Imagine that you are hugging a large beach ball as you bring your arms into a closed hug position **(Photo P)**. Keep your elbows lifted, and pull your shoulder blades down your back to relax your shoulders. Tap the tip of both of your little fingers into your palms five times, followed by your ring fingers five times **(Photo Q)**, middle fingers five times, index fingers five times, and thumbs five times. Repeat the sequence with four taps with each of your fingers and thumbs, then three, then two, and finish with one tap into your palm with each of your fingers and thumbs.

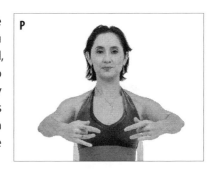

Why It's Beneficial

Clara Pilates developed the Pre-Pilates Castanets exercise to help with painful rheumatoid arthritis in her hands. Developing mobility in your fingers is more important now than ever. People are beginning to develop tight hands because of time spent with electronic devices. The Castanets exercise strengthens the arms and loosens up tight joints in the fingers.

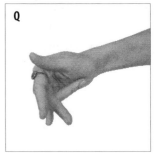

Eventually

The same exercise can be performed with more flamenco flavor by changing the carriage of the arms during the exercise. The arms can lift to frame the face **(Photo R)**, they can open to the side, and the arms can stay low with the hands just slightly behind the body. For even more flamenco style, the exercise can transition from sitting down to standing on both feet, to standing on one leg with the other leg reaching forward so that the front leg is slightly bent and the heel of the front foot is raised above the floor.

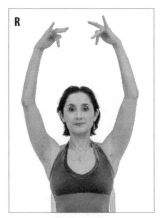

GOING BEYOND PRE-PILATES FOR THE HANDS

HAIR TIE EXERCISE

Getting Started

Sit on the front edge of a chair with your feet parallel and apart on the floor. Place your forearms on your thighs, with your wrists and hands a few inches in front of your knees. Resting your forearms on your thighs provides greater isolation and stability for your wrists and helps you focus on just your fingers.

Loop a thin hair tie (average size is about 7cm long) around the thumb, just under the thumbnail. To keep the hair tie from flying off the fingers or sliding down to the base of the fingers, twist the hair tie with the index finger of your opposite hand and leave just enough room at the top for another loop. Put the loop over the tip of the index finger on the hand that already has the thumb in the hair tie.

Push your feet into the floor as you lift your bellybutton away from the floor. With your powerhouse engaged and your shoulders even, move your index finger away from your thumb and stretch the hair tie for the count of three seconds. To help isolate the other parts of the hand as you stretch the hair tie, imagine that your finger is a door that opens and closes from a hinge at the base of your working finger. The movement can be performed 3 times on each of the fingers of both hands, or on just one finger of each hand. **Photos S-T**

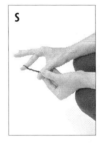 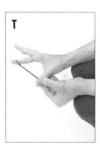

Why It's Beneficial

The Hair Tie Exercise is inspired by the exercise performed with the Hand Tens-O-Meter apparatus, also known as the Magic Square finger apparatus. The Hand Tens-O-Meter resembles the Pilates Toe Corrector, but the loops for the fingers are on the opposite sides of the spring. When using the Hand-Tens-O-Meter, the exertion happens when the fingers press toward the thumb. In contrast, in the Hair Tie Exercise the exertion happens as the fingers stretch away from the thumb. Doing the Hair Tie Exercise is a good way to combat cramps in the hands due to overuse from typing, using mobile devices, writing, playing musical instruments, and sports.

Finger exercises with the twisted hair tie strengthen the muscles used to move the fingers. Fingers do not contain muscles for finger movement. The only muscles in the fingers are attached to hair follicles that can make the hairs on the fingers stand out straight. Tendons attached to the bones in our fingers are also attached to muscles in the palms of our hands, and to muscles in our forearms. This exercise works the muscles in the palm of the hand and in the forearm.

Injuries to the upper extremities that require finger splints, shoulder slings, or arm casts lead to weakened muscles. This is an excellent exercise for people who have received a doctor's approval to start strengthening exercises after recovery from upper extremity injuries. This exercise helps reawaken the muscles that move the fingers. It is particularly useful for strengthening fingers that have healed from fractures and dislocation.

Tips

When performing the Hair Tie exercise, make sure that you maintain long wrists and isolate your thumb as you move the fingertip in the other end of the hair tie. Securing the hair tie over your thumb with your other hand will help to stabilize your thumb, keep your thumb in line with your joint, and avoid fly away hair ties.

Eventually
When you have good control and can isolate your thumbs and maintain long wrists, you can perform this exercise without resting your forearms on your thighs.

SAND BAG MOVEMENT WITH A ROLLING PIN
Getting Started
Stand in Pilates stance or another stance appropriate for your body and pull your bellybutton in and up. Your weight should be light on your heels with your thighs pulled up and your knees soft. Hold the handles of a rolling pin with your fingers on top and your thumbs underneath. Lift your arms in front of you with your arms slightly rounded. Imagine that your elbows are resting on an imaginary tabletop. Remember to keep your collarbones open and your shoulder blades down.

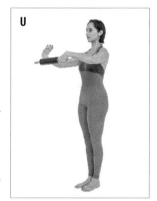

To begin the movement, release your grip on one handle and spread your fingers as you draw your fingertips back. The wrist of the other hand, still gripping the handle, rolls forward **(Photo U)**. Continue to alternate hands, and then reverse the direction.

As you roll the handles of the rolling pin forward, imagine that your fingers are digging through sand each time you release the handle and draw your fingertips toward the ceiling. As you roll the handles of the rolling pin backward, imagine that you are revving a motorcycle. Do the forward motion 16 times followed by the backward motion 16 times.

Why It's Beneficial
This exercise mimics the hand movement used to unwind and wind a long string on the wooden dowel of the Sand Bag apparatus. Eliminating the string and the three-pound bag of sand makes the exercise available to more people. It works the fingers, wrists, forearms, and upper arms. It also emphasizes good posture and develops coordination.
Tips
Remember to keep your elbows even and isolate your arms as you move your hands. The handles of the rolling pin should not dip as you do this exercise. Keep the effort in your powerhouse and relax your shoulders as you grip the rolling pin. Unlike most Pilates exercises, the thumbs do not stay on the same side as the fingers in this exercise.

Eventually
In time, you can move beyond 1 set of 16 wrist rolls forward followed by 16 wrist rolls backward. The goal is to keep the wrists moving for 3 continuous sets.

PRE-PILATES FOR THE ARMS

INTRODUCTION
Fractures in the upper arms and forearms are common. One reason is that an outstretched arm/hand is usually the first point of contact in a fall. When my mother was in her sixties, she fell and broke her upper arm. At the hospital, it became clear that surgery was unavoidable. She now has titanium rods holding her humerus bone together.

Elbow injuries are also common. Elbow pain can have many causes including arthritis, tendonitis, bursitis, sprains and strains, fractures, and dislocations. I had a brief experience with elbow pain and in my situation the Pre-Pilates exercises were very helpful.

The Finger Flicks, Wrist Twirls/Floreo, and Castanet exercises, are very good for strengthening the forearms and upper arms. See the Hands section in this chapter for details.

SHAKING OUT THE ARMS

Getting Started

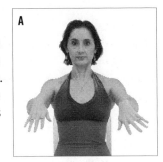

Sit on the edge of a chair and plant your feet on the floor. With your powerhouse muscles activated, lift your arms out in front of you at shoulder height. Begin to shake out your hands and arms and then stop to feel the tingling sensation there. Imagine that you have just washed your hands and have no towel with which to dry your hands. You need to shake your hands vigorously to shake off the excess water. **Photo A**

Why It's Beneficial

Depending on the way you do it, the Pre-Pilates version of Shaking Out the Arms can achieve different goals. It can be used as a warm-up to get the blood circulating in the hands and arms. It can promote relaxation in the arms after an exercise for arm strength. It can also be used as an invigorating energy builder to re-center your focus.

In the Dead Bug exercise, which usually follows the Side Leg Series on the mat, the student lies on his back and extends his limbs toward the ceiling, gently shaking them out. Keeping the limbs above the heart draws the blood toward the powerhouse. In the Shaking Out the Arms exercise, your arms do not go above shoulder level to drain blood out of your arms, and your arms do not dangle by the sides of your body to draw blood into the arms. The arms extend forward at shoulder level, and you are either seated or standing. This promotes a general circulation of the blood.

Eventually

For a variation of this exercise that sharpens the mental focus, stand and count backwards in even numbers from eight. Shake your right arm to each count (8,6,4,2), then your left arm, and then both arms together. Repeat counting odd numbers from seven. Perform one set with even numbers and one set with odd numbers.

Applications Outside the Pilates Studio

When I was a young dancer recuperating from a broken leg and sprained ankle, I worked with Igor Burdenko, creator of the Burdenko Method. Much like Joe Pilates, who used springs to provide both resistance and support in rehabilitative and conditioning exercises, Igor created exercises that use water for both resistance and support. Among the many exercises Igor taught me, one of my favorites was a simple warm-up exercise in which I shook my arms and legs in the deep end of the pool while using a water belt for buoyancy. I loved the way it released tension and promoted circulation in my body. As a dancer I also used to shake out my limbs to help calm my nerves before stepping onstage.

HUG WITH FISTS

Getting Started

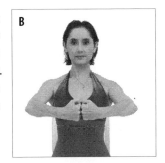

To perform this exercise while seated, sit on the edge of a chair with your feet together or parallel and apart on the floor. Wrap your arms around an imaginary basket and make fists. Activate your powerhouse muscles, then activate your arm muscles by pressing the knuckles of your fists into each other for three seconds. To find the correct shape in the arms and wrists, imagine that you are holding a cup in each hand and clicking the cups together on each repetition. Perform up to 3 times. **Photo B**

Why It's Beneficial

This is a good Pre-Pilates exercise for building strength in the chest and upper arms. Many of the Pre-Pilates exercises for the hands also have the added benefit of working the arms. But in this exercise, the entire focus is on the arms. It was one of the first exercises I gave my son when a broken bone in his upper arm had healed completely.

Tips

When Romana taught me the Pumping exercise on the Electric Chair, she had me wrap my arms around the pipes/shovels of the chair. She told me to imagine that I was creating electricity in my arms and body in order to get the pedal moving. Inspired by that image, I like to imagine that I am creating an electrical charge throughout my arms and chest as I press my fists together.

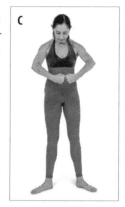

This is one of the few Pre-Pilates exercises that can be performed in three postures: supine, seated, and standing. It is more common to learn the Hug with Fists while seated or standing. If you have trouble keeping your collar bones open as you draw your fists together, you can do the exercise lying on your back, with your legs bent and your feet resting on the mat. Press your fists into one another as you pull your bellybutton down into the mat. To open your chest, think of spreading your upper back on the mat as you draw your knuckles together.

Eventually

The Hug with Fists eventually progresses into the archival Hug/Arm Circle Combination. See Joe's Archival Routine chapter for details. **Photo C**

GOING BEYOND PRE-PILATES FOR THE ARMS

WALL SERIES: PEEL DOWN

Getting Started

Stand with your back against the wall and your feet away from the wall. Bring your chin to your chest and begin to peel one vertebra at a time away from the wall as you bend forward. As you peel your spine from the wall, breathe out. After you complete the peel down, imagine that you are a rag doll with your head and arms hanging freely. Breathe naturally, with your stomach muscles engaged, as your hanging arms and hands draw five little circles away from your midline, and five little circles toward your midline. As your arms dangle, imagine that your arms are pendulums moving in tiny circles. Once the circles are completed, roll your spine up against the wall as you breathe in. Perform 2-3 times.

Why It's Beneficial

The Peel Down incorporates breathing, spinal articulation, and inversion, making it a good choice for ending a lesson. At the suggestion of my son's orthopedist, I gave my son the Peel Down from the Wall Series after he broke his arm. With his arms hanging like a ragdoll's, he made a pendulum motion in a very small range, which helped to avoid stiffness in his elbow from the many hours spent in his arm sling each day. The pendulum motion also promoted the remodeling of his humerus bone, which had been thirty degrees out of alignment after the break.

The Peel Down can be performed on its own, or as the second exercise in the Wall Series. All the exercises from the Wall Series strengthen the arms and shoulders and develop symmetry of movement in the arms. Consult *Pilates: An Interactive Workbook* to view the entire series.

Tips

All the exercises from the Wall Series can be performed with the addition of weights. When you are ready to add weights, be sure not to hold more than three pounds in each hand. **Photos D-H**

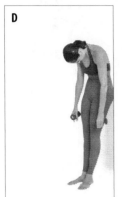 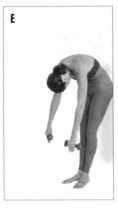 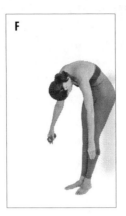 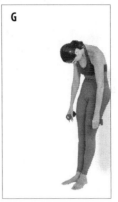 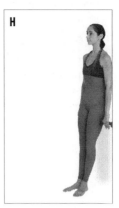

As you roll your spine up against the wall, slide your tailbone down as you lift your bellybutton in opposition. You can think of a paint roller sliding up a wall as you roll up through your spine.

Eventually

Instead of moving your heels away from the wall to perform the Peel Down, keep your heels against the wall and try to reach for your toes as you peel your back from the wall. Perform 2-3 times.

STANDING WEIGHTS SERIES: STANDING CURLS

Getting Started

Stand in Pilates stance, or another stance that is appropriate for your body. Extend your arms long by your sides, palms facing forward. Keep your elbows by your sides as you bring your fingertips up toward your shoulders and back down by your sides. Perform 3-5 times.

Why It's Beneficial

The Standing Weights Series is designed to strengthen the arms. The Standing Curls exercise is especially import-ant for people who have had an arm immobilized in a sling or cast. It helps to work out stiffness in the elbow joint and regain mobility. The Standing Curls also strengthen the biceps and the forearms. Consult *Pilates: An Interactive Workbook* to view all the exercises from the Standing Weights Series.

Tips

The key to success in all of the Standing Weights exercises is to perform them with resistance. The resistance has nothing to do with whether or not you hold weights, and everything to do with the intention you put into the exercise. One of the best ways to get a sense of creating resistance as you move your arms in the Standing Weights series is to imagine that you are performing the arm movements under water. As your arms move away from your midline, imagine that your hands are pushing water away. As your arms move toward your midline, imagine that your hands are pulling water toward you. Learning the Standing Weights series without holding weights makes it easier to focus on creating resistance and is helpful to people who hyperextend their elbows.

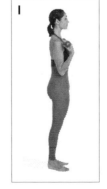 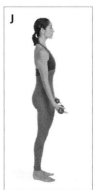

When the time comes to add weights, be sure not to exceed three pounds in each hand. **Photos I-J**

Eventually
To work the wrists, you can follow each arm curl with a wrist extension. Stretch your arms long by your sides, and bend your wrists so that your fingertips extend away from your body, palms facing the floor and fingertips reaching up. **Photo K**

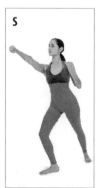
K

MAGIC CIRCLE ARM SERIES: ARMS IN FRONT AND BEHIND
Why It's Beneficial
The Shuffling the Ball exercise is a modified version of the Standing Arm Exercises with the Magic Circle. It improves posture while working the arms and developing coordination.

Tips
Some people sacrifice the length in their arms when they attempt to pulse the Magic Circle between their hands. Letting the arms shorten shifts the focus from the powerhouse to the arms. Instead of using the Magic Circle, you can quickly transfer a basketball, volleyball, or soccer ball back and forth between your hands.

Getting Started
Stand in a stance appropriate for your body, holding a basketball, volleyball or soccer ball. With your powerhouse lifted, extend your arms in front of your waist and transfer the ball back and forth between your two hands. Maintain long arms and fingers as you shuffle the ball back and forth. **Photo L**

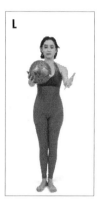
L

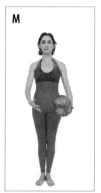
M

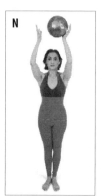
N

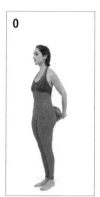
O

Once you gain confidence shuffling the ball at waist level, try to shuffle the ball between your hands with your arms down in front of your thighs **(Photo M)**. Next, try to shuffle the ball between your hands with your arms reaching toward the ceiling **(Photo N)**. You can also try to shuffle the ball back and forth with your arms behind you **(Photo O)**. Make sure that you keep your fingertips reaching toward the floor and your collarbones open.

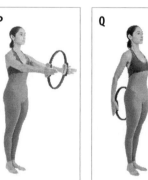
P
Q

Eventually
Once you are able to shuffle the ball back and forth without shortening your arms, you can replace the ball with the Magic Circle. **Photos P and Q**

OTHER EXERCISES THAT GO BEYOND PRE-PILATES FOR THE ARMS

JOE'S STANDING ARM EXERCISES
Joe Pilates created a series of standing exercises for the upper body that are not performed with weights. The Archival Ninety Degrees Side **(Photo R)**, Archival Side Bends, Hug/Arm Circle Combination, Archival Shave and Archival Boxing **(Photo S)** are good exercises for strengthening the arms beyond the Pre-Pilates level. For more details on these exercises, see the Joe's Archival Routine chapter starting on page 82.

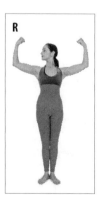
R

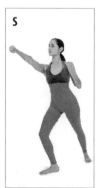
S

PRE-PILATES FOR THE SHOULDERS

INTRODUCTION

Well before I had my own children, I went to the home of a student to meet her newborn son. She was the first student to do Pilates with me throughout her pregnancy. In my effort to keep my first "Pilates baby" happy and comfortable, I failed to notice the tension I was storing in my shoulders, until I felt a minor shoulder ache later that evening. As more "Pilates babies" were born, I noticed a recurring complaint of shoulder pain among these new parents. I realized that they were developing overuse injuries in their shoulders from holding and/or nursing their babies.

When I became a mother, I was determined to avoid the same fate. I discovered a pillow that is designed to take pressure off your back and shoulders as you hold and/or nurse your baby. I affectionately referred to it as my "baby tutu" because it wrapped around my waist and stuck out like a ballerina costume after being hooked together in the back. It saved my shoulders from a lot of strain. I recommend the pillow to all my expectant mothers and fathers. Yes, dads of newborns complain of shoulder pain too. I also did my best to use my body awareness and not favor one side of my body as I held my baby. It was a challenge that only became harder when I had my second baby 22 months later.

My effort to avoid shoulder pain paid off when my children were babies, but a dozen years later I injured my left shoulder lifting a concrete planter out of the trunk of my car. I have to be very conscientious about my range of movement, I avoid abrupt movements, and I am extremely careful about how much weight I put on my left shoulder. In the Pilates studio I have struck a delicate balance, doing exercises that maintain both flexibility and strength in my shoulder without aggravating my injury. The Pre-Pilates exercises for the shoulder have been invaluable as I monitor my progress.

SHRUGS

Getting Started
Learn the Shrugs in a seated position with your legs bent at ninety degrees and feet on the floor. Engage your stomach, bottom, and inner thigh muscles before beginning the movement. With your arms long by your sides, simultaneously inhale as you lift your shoulders to your ears. Keep your shoulders raised for three counts as you hold your breath. Next, take one count to gently let your shoulders relax as you breathe out. Perform 3-5 times. **Photos A-B**

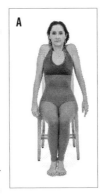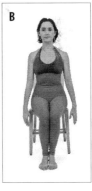

Why It's Beneficial
The Shoulder Shrugs promote relaxation. Do them first thing in the morning, and throughout the day, to rid the body of unwanted shoulder tension.

Tips
Lifting the shoulders up and down is a good exercise for teaching us about the muscles that move the shoulder blades. By moving the shoulders from one extreme to the other, we learn to feel the difference between contracting the upper trapezius and levator scapulae muscles, when the shoulders lift, and contracting the lower trapezius muscles when the shoulders press down.

Eventually
With practice, the Shrugs can be performed standing, while holding a one-pound weight in each hand. Let the one-pound weights gently pull the tension out of your shoulders. Holding something in the hands while performing the Shrugs will remind you to keep your shoulders relaxed when you hold things.

SHOULDER ROLLS

Getting Started

Start in a seated position, with your legs bent at ninety degrees and your feet on the floor. With your powerhouse muscles activated, pull your shoulder blades toward each other as you open your collarbones. Then, lift your shoulders to your ears and bring your shoulders forward as you open your upper back. Perform 3 times and reverse 3 times. **Photos C-F**

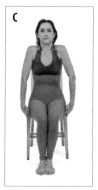 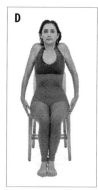 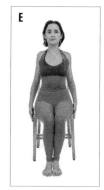 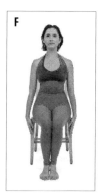

Why It's Beneficial

The Shoulder Rolls improve mobility in the shoulder joints. Keeping the shoulders limber and free of tension also benefits the neck. Make sure that you perform the Shoulder Rolls slowly and with control. Like the Pre-Pilates Shrugs, the Shoulder Rolls can be done first thing in the morning or throughout the day to relieve tension.

Tips

Be sure that the Shoulder Rolls move from back to front on the first 3 rolls so that the reverse rolls finish with the shoulders back and the chest open. Rolling the shoulders back engages the rhomboid muscles, which are under the middle trapezius muscles. The rhomboid muscles are attached from the spine to the inside of the shoulder blades, the scapulae, and help to retract the shoulders. Strengthening the middle trapezius and rhomboid muscles is important for developing good posture.

Eventually

To check for evenness in the shoulders, the Shoulder Rolls can be performed standing while holding a rolling pin. Be sure that the rolling pin is always parallel to the floor as the shoulders roll.

SPIDER

Getting Started

Stand facing a wall at about a forearm's distance away, with your powerhouse muscles engaged. Your elbows are in your frame, touching your sides. You place your fingertips on the wall at waist level. Create a dome shape with your hands, fingertips touching the wall with the palms lifted away from the wall. Using the pads of your fingertips, not thumbs, you try to climb the wall with the fingers of each hand moving in unison: index fingers, followed by middle fingers, ring fingers, and little fingers. Repeat the pattern all the way up to your limit. Imagine that your fingertips have suction cups that stick to the wall with each step. Remember to slide your shoulder blades down your back with each step of the fingertip.

Once your arms reach the maximum height possible without causing pain, walk a little closer to the wall if you can, or you may stay where you are. Hold this position for a few seconds as you focus on lengthening your spine, sliding your shoulder blades down your back, and pulling your ribs in. To finish, you will step back and let your fingertips slide down the wall. Perform up to 3 times. **Photo G**

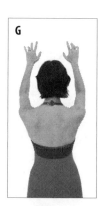

Why It's Beneficial

The Spider exercise is designed to increase the range of motion in the shoulder joint. It is good for people who have had an arm in a cast or sling, and are ready to regain their range of motion. It helps to prevent or rehabilitate a frozen shoulder.

Keeping It Real

Although my son's broken humerus bone got stronger after its fracture, he developed a frozen shoulder from his arm being in a sling for eight weeks. The Spider exercise was an extremely challenging exercise for him when he got his doctor's approval to work on regaining shoulder flexibility. As he lifted his arm, he compensated for his lack of shoulder flexibility by arching his back, letting his ribs stick out, and straining his neck. I did not let him resume his sports activities until he could perform the Spider exercise with the back of his neck long and relaxed, his shoulders plugged into his shoulder joints, and his ribs closed.

Eventually

For a more intense stretch in the shoulders and chest, perform the Spider with your elbows open, similar to the Shave exercise position. Since the elbows move outside the frame of the body in this variation of the Spider, do not add it too soon. When the time is right, it will improve lateral arm movement, which is often the hardest range of motion to regain in the shoulder joint after a shoulder injury.

Stand with your toes as close to the wall as possible, your head turned to one side, your elbows pointing away from your midline, and your fingertips on the wall. Your arms should feel weightless as your arms hang from the imaginary suction cups on your fingertips. After climbing to the maximum height possible without pain, pay attention to lengthening your spine as you pull your abdominal muscles in and up. Let the hands "drip" down the wall to finish. Repeat with the other ear facing the wall. Perform 2 times. **Photos H-J**

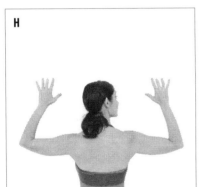 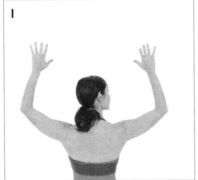 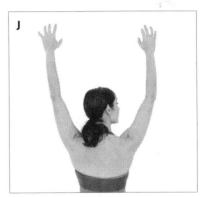

GOING BEYOND PRE-PILATES FOR THE SHOULDERS

PILATES PUSH-UPS ON THE WALL

Getting Started

Place your hands on the wall directly in front of your shoulders and walk your feet back so that your feet are slightly beyond your arms' distance from the wall. Keep your feet flat on the floor in a stance that suits your body. Pilates stance is ideal, but feet together or parallel and apart are also good. Push your hips slightly forward into a firm diagonal line. Your body creates one long line from the crown of your head, through your hips, and into your heels. Remember to pull your stomach in, hug your inner thighs toward your midline, and squeeze your seat. Keeping the arms straight, hold the position for at least three seconds.

When you have sufficient strength holding the plank shape, add the Pilates Push-Ups. Be sure that your elbows stay within the frame of your body as your arms bend. If you can maintain the integrity of your plank shape, take your elbows all the way to the wall. Do two push-ups and on the third push-up, keep your arms bent for three counts. Perform 2 sets of 3 Pilates Push-Ups. **Photos K-L**

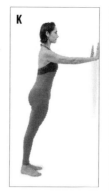 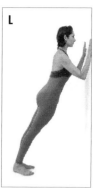

As you progress, you can perform Pilates Push-Ups on the Wall with your feet on the half toe. Perform 2 sets of 3 Pilates Push-Ups on the half toe.

Why It's Beneficial
Pilates Push-ups develop powerhouse strength as well as strength in the chest, shoulders, and triceps. Keeping your upper body elevated on the wall, as opposed to putting the hands down on the floor, is a safe way to introduce Pilates Push-Ups to people who are still developing powerhouse and upper body strength.

Tips
The most important part of a push-up is the plank position. Romana told me to imagine that I was a "solid piece of steel from head to heel" in the plank shape.

Eventually
To work one side at a time, do one-handed Pilates Push-Ups on the wall. Be sure to move your working arm in slightly on the wall, so that it is between your midline and your working shoulder. Your other arm wraps around your waist. The half toe position can be distracting during one-handed Pilates Push-Ups, so keep your feet flat on the floor for this variation. Perform 3 Pilates Push-Ups on the weak side, repeat on the stronger side, and do an extra set on the weaker side. **Photos M-N**

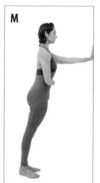 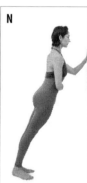

PILATES PUSH-UPS ON THE FLOOR
Why It's Beneficial
As your powerhouse and upper body strength increase, add exercises with your hands supporting more of your body weight. Pilates Push-ups on the floor develop powerhouse strength, as well as strength in the chest, shoulders, and triceps.

Getting Started
Start with the kneeling plank on the floor if you have not developed enough powerhouse and upper body strength to support your own weight safely. A kneeling plank creates a long line from the crown of the head, through the hips, to the knees, with the shins elevated off the mat and ankles crossed.

Once the kneeling plank has been mastered, do the final plank position on the mat. When first learning this plank shape with straight legs, begin kneeling on the mat with your hands under your shoulders and fingers facing forward. Your arms are perpendicular to the floor, with your shoulders directly above your hands. Remember to keep your arms long with soft elbows. Next, extend one leg behind you on the half-toe with your heel aligned directly over the ball of your foot. Once you have a feel for the long line with one foot on the ground, take the second leg back and try to hold the plank for three counts. **Photo O**

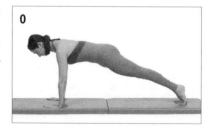

Tips

The most important part of a push-up is the plank position. If you do not engage your powerhouse, your hips may drop and your plank will resemble a wet noodle. If you try to relieve pressure in your powerhouse, you may lift your hips so that you resemble an inchworm. A safe push-up position must have all three parts of the powerhouse activated: the stomach, the bottom, and the inner thighs. To create the ideal plank shape, think of creating a C-curve in the low back, while pulling your chest forward.

Eventually

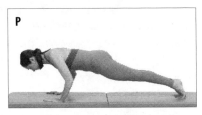

Once you have developed a strong plank position on the mat, you can add the Pilates Push-Ups. Begin standing in a Pilates stance, with your powerhouse engaged and your arms reaching toward the ceiling. Roll through your spine and fold in half with your hands on the floor, and walk your hands forward into the plank position. Perform one to three Pilates Push-ups with your elbows in your frame **(Photo P)**. Remember that you need to push your body directly *up*, not back, in order to keep your shoulders over your wrists as you complete each Pilates Push-up. To come out of the Pilates Push-Up, bring your chin to your chest and lift your ribs and bellybutton toward the ceiling before walking your hands back toward your feet. Roll up your spine and finish the way you began, with your arms reaching up. Perform 1-3 sets of 3 Pilates Push-Ups.

L-SHAPE AGAINST THE WALL

Getting Started

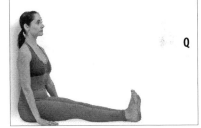

This exercise is performed with the hands positioned on the floor at a measurement equal to your leg length from the wall. To find your leg's distance from the wall, sit on the floor with your back to the wall and your legs extended forward. **Photo Q**

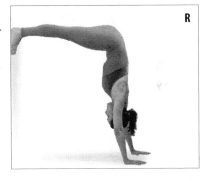

Stand up where your feet were while you were seated, and position your hands on the floor by your feet. With your head tucked in and your powerhouse lifted, you walk your feet back to the wall and up it, into an "L" shape with your torso perpendicular to the floor and your legs parallel to the floor. Hold for three counts. **Photo R**

Why It's Beneficial

The L-Shape Against the Wall strengthens the arms, shoulders, and upper back and stabilizes the powerhouse muscles. It reverses the blood flow toward the brain, which can provide an energizing effect. The elements of fun and inversion make the L-Shape an exciting final exercise for a workout.

Tips

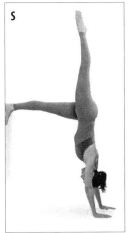

Remember to activate your stomach, bottom, and inner thigh muscles to avoid wiggles. Tuck your head in to maintain proper form. Imagine that you are pushing the floor away as your hands press firmly into the floor.

Eventually

When you are ready, lift one leg toward the ceiling as you hold the L-shape in your torso and supporting leg **(Photo S)**. After returning your foot to the wall, lift the other leg. To come out of the exercise walk your feet down the wall and forward on the floor toward your hands. Roll up to standing to complete the movement.

OTHER EXERCISES THAT GO BEYOND PRE-PILATES FOR THE SHOULDERS

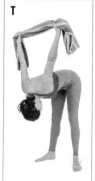

WAKE-UP EXERCISES FOR THE UPPER BODY

Romana gave upper body exercises performed with a towel held between the hands as part of the "Exercises For Businessmen" routine. These exercises are good for people with stiff but healthy shoulders. They work the upper body, increase shoulder flexibility, stretch the chest muscles, and develop powerhouse control as the arms move. These exercises involve a large range of motion, so be sure that you are ready to go beyond the Pre-Pilates moves for the shoulders before you add these exercises to your lesson plan. See the Wake-Up Exercises chapter starting on page 63 for details. **Photo T**

CARTWHEELS

For the ultimate shoulder strengthening exercise, people with healthy shoulders can use the hands to support the full weight of the body. See the Cartwheel exercise on pages 110-111 in Romana's Standing Exercises chapter for details. **Photo U**

PRE-PILATES FOR THE NECK

INTRODUCTION

I have a delicate neck. The first time I sprained my neck, I was pregnant with my son. I couldn't even lift my head off my pillow without the help of my hands and moving it was extremely painful. Because I was pregnant, I couldn't take any anti-inflammatory medication to ease my discomfort. I did acupuncture and Pre-Pilates neck exercises to increase circulation to the area until the pain subsided. My neck is delicate because I used to push myself to do an acrobatic-like Pilates move before I had the necessary upper body strength to keep the pressure off my neck. I no longer let my ego take priority over my wellbeing, but it took time and multiple neck sprains to gain that wisdom. I was once told that the higher an injury is on your body, the more debilitating it can be, and from my own experience, I wholeheartedly agree.

In Pilates, the neck is considered the second powerhouse, because it is responsible for supporting the head, which is the heaviest part of the body. It takes most babies a month to develop the muscle strength necessary to lift the head up, four months to hold the head up in a seated position, and six months to acquire steady strength and control in the neck muscles.

People spend a lot of time sticking their necks forward toward their computer screens and hunched over their mobile devices. The effect of technology overload on the neck has been given the name "tech neck." Pre-Pilates neck exercises stretch the neck muscles and improve range of motion. Since shoulder tension and neck tension are usually linked, the Pre-Pilates Shoulder Shrugs and Shoulder Rolls are also good for limbering the neck. These exercises can serve as an ideal warm-up before using mobile devices, and as a good cool down after finishing with them. Aside from doing Pre-Pilates exercises for the neck, try to limit your tech time and take frequent breaks during time spent on these devices. The head weighs 12 pounds. Add to that the feeling of an extra ten pounds for every inch out of alignment, and you are begging for neck pain.

NOSE CIRCLES AND NECK SEMI-CIRCLES

Getting Started

Sit or stand with your powerhouse lifted. Without letting your nose point to the sky, use the tip of your nose to draw a very small circle, no bigger than a tennis ball. Perform 3 circles and then reverse the direction for 3 repetitions.

Why It's Beneficial

In Pilates, full neck circles are never performed. Rolling the head backward can inhibit blood flow and compress the spine. Tracing circles no bigger than a tennis ball, or drawing half circles with the tip of the nose in a slow and controlled manner, are the safest ways to stretch the neck.

Tips

To fully grasp how hard the neck muscles work to support the weight of the head, you can compare the weight of the head on the neck to a fish bowl balancing on a fingertip.

Eventually

For a deeper neck stretch, use your nose to trace a semi-circle. Starting with your gaze straight ahead, turn your head to one shoulder. As your chin rolls across your chest toward the other shoulder, imagine that you are using your nose to draw a smiley face. Finish the semi-circle looking straight ahead. Perform one more semi-circle starting in the opposite direction. **Photos A-F**

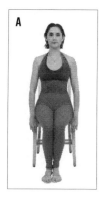 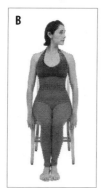 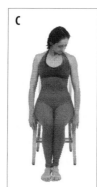 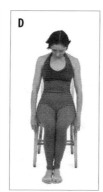 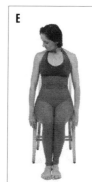 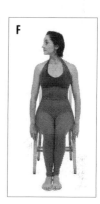

NECK ROTATION

Getting Started

Sit or stand with your focus on your powerhouse, then check your neck placement. Make sure that you are not sticking your chin out. Your head is retracted back toward the centerline, but not beyond. To correct forward head posture, think of drawing your jawline back.

After taking a deep breath in, rotate your chin toward one shoulder as you breathe out for three seconds and repeat to the other side. Remember to keep your movements slow and controlled. Without moving your shoulders, try to see what is behind you as you turn your head.

Why It's Beneficial

Turning the head side to side promotes neck flexibility and relieves tension in the neck. The Neck Rotation exercise is a helpful exercise to do throughout the day to keep everyday stresses from invading the neck and shoulders.

Tips

I like to have my students perform the Neck Rotation exercise with the arms raised just in front of the ears, thumbs interlaced if possible. Raising the arms encourages an extra lift in the powerhouse. The added lift in the powerhouse improves posture. Better posture improves the range of movement in the neck. Try this exercise in a slouched position and you will feel the reduced range of motion in the neck. In addition to the lift in the powerhouse, elevating the arms tends to open the collarbones. When the collarbones are lifted, tension is released in the chest. The shoulder blades are then in a more favorable position for the neck rotation. Perform 4 times, alternating sides. **Photo G**

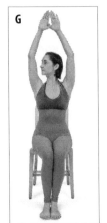

Eventually
If you are lifting your head off the mat in the Matwork series for exercises like the Hundred and Series of Five, you can rotate your neck in the supine position between exercises, as a way to keep tension out of your neck. Look at the mat with your left eye when turning your head toward the right shoulder. Look at the mat with your right eye when turning your head toward the left shoulder.

It is also beneficial to turn the head side to side as a means of checking the head and neck alignment in the headrest, after lying down on the Reformer. Remember to turn your head slowly, because if you are not centered between the two Reformer shoulder blocks, your chin might hit a shoulder block as you turn your head.

Performing the Neck Rotation is also helpful when standing in an inverted position, such as the Peel Down from the Wall Series, or the second part of the Backbend on the Ladder Barrel. To make sure you are keeping your neck relaxed while standing with your upper body folded forward, try to shake your head, as if to say "no."

EAR TO SHOULDER
Getting Started
Engage all three parts of your powerhouse: stomach, bottom, and inner thigh muscles, as you sit or stand. Your gaze remains straight ahead throughout the exercise. Inhale with your head centered over your midline, and gently exhale as you bend your head toward one shoulder. On the next inhalation, center your head again, and then breathe out as your head bends toward the other shoulder. Hold the stretch for three seconds before centering the head. Perform 4 times, alternating sides. **Photo H**

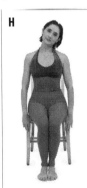

Why It's Beneficial
Bending the head to the side as the ear drops toward the shoulder is a very good neck stretch targeting the trapezius muscles. It is an excellent exercise for people who are over-contracting their trapezius muscles repeatedly while using computers and mobile devices.

Tips
Remember not to let the shoulder lift; bring the ear toward the shoulder.

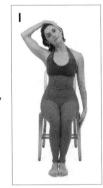

Perform this exercise in front of a mirror so that you can monitor tilting your head without rotating it as you bring your ear to your shoulder. As you bend your neck toward your shoulder, remember to keep your arms long by your sides, with your fingertips actively reaching down to the floor. When the arms, especially the arm on the side of the neck being stretched, are actively reaching to the floor, the stretch is more productive.

Eventually
For a deeper trapezius stretch, place your hand on your head to achieve a deeper stretch. As your head bends toward your right shoulder, wrap your right arm around your head to deepen the stretch. As your head bends toward your left shoulder, wrap your left arm around your head to deepen the stretch. **Photo I**

GOING BEYOND PRE-PILATES FOR THE NECK

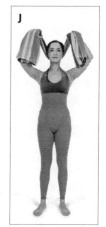

ASSISTED NECK STRETCH WITH THE TOWEL

The Assisted Neck Stretch promotes circulation in the neck and the towel provides additional stretch, support, and gentle traction. See page 68 in the Wake-Up Exercises chapter. **Photo J**

MAGIC CIRCLE NECK EXERCISES WITH THE HANDS

The Magic Circle exercises for the neck can be used to strengthen and/or stretch the neck. See the Magic Circle chapter in *Pilates: An Interactive Workbook* for details. But for a gentler stretch, replace the Magic Circle with your hands:

MAGIC CIRCLE NECK EXERCISES WITH THE HANDS: THUMBS UNDER THE CHIN

Tips

There is a temptation to stick the chin out when using the Magic Circle under the chin. Another option is to use the hands, rather than the circle, for resistance.

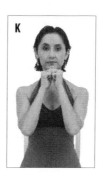
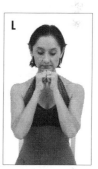

Getting Started

This exercise can be performed seated or standing. Activate your power-house muscles, make two fists, and place your thumbs under your chin. With your hands resisting the pressure of your chin, gently press your chin into your hands. **Photo K**

Eventually

After you are used to resisting the pressure of your chin with your thumbs, lower your head slightly as you press your chin toward your chest. **Photo L**

Why It's Beneficial

This exercise strengthens the front of the neck. The additional movement of the head lowering slightly also provides a stretch in the back of the neck.

MAGIC CIRCLE NECK EXERCISES WITH THE HANDS: FOREHEAD

Tips

Instead of putting the cushion of the Magic Circle on your forehead, you can use your hands for resistance.

Getting Started

You can learn this in a seated position with your hands stacked on your forehead and your elbows lifted. You press your hands gently into your forehead, resisting the pressure of your hands. Press and hold for three seconds. Perform up to 3 times. **Photo M**

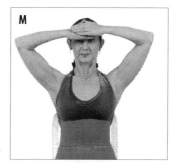

To release neck tension, follow this neck strengthening exercise with the Neck Rotation exercise on pages 53-54 **(Photo G)**.

Why It's Beneficial

This exercise strengthens the neck. It is not intended for people with delicate necks.

Eventually
When you are ready, you can try this exercise standing. Keep your weight forward on the balls of your feet as you press your hands gently into your forehead.

To release neck tension, follow this neck strengthening exercise with the Chest Expansion exercise on page 57 **(Photos P-T)**.

MAGIC CIRCLE NECK EXERCISES WITH THE HANDS: BACK OF THE HEAD

Why It's Beneficial
This exercise strengthens the back of the neck when the hands are stacked behind the head and stretches the neck when the hands are positioned under the base of the skull.

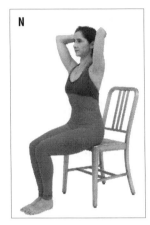

Getting Started
To strengthen the back of the neck, stack your hands behind your head and gently press the back of your head into your hands, resisting the pressure. Make sure that your chin does not lift. Press and hold for three counts. Perform up to 3 times. **Photo N**

To stretch the back of the neck, separate your hands and position your palms, in the area near the finger pad, at the base of your skull. While maintaining an elongated line in the back of your neck, use your hands to create traction as you pull up at the base of your skull. This is a good way to release neck and shoulder tension. Perform up to 3 times.

Tips
When the hands are stacked behind the head, fingers are not interlaced. Interlaced fingers are always avoided in Pilates because that tends to put extra tension in the shoulders.

Eventually
You can incorporate this exercise into the Flat Back from the Short Box Series on the Reformer and the Neck Pull from the Intermediate Matwork. Consult *Pilates: An Interactive Workbook* for details.

MAGIC CIRCLE NECK EXERCISES WITH THE HANDS: SIDE OF THE HEAD

Tips
Instead of putting the cushion of the Magic Circle on the side of the head, use your hands for resistance. Keeping the head in line with the midline of the body is challenging in this exercise, so perform it in front of a mirror and watch for alignment.

Getting Started
Seated or standing, put the heel of your hand on the side of your head, just above your ear. As you press your hand gently into your head, try to keep your head centered above the midline, resisting the pressure. Press and hold for three counts. Perform up to 3 times on each side. **Photo O**

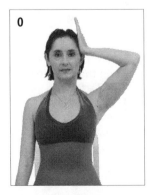

Why It's Beneficial
This exercise strengthens the sides of the neck.

Eventually

Eventually, you can combine these isometric Magic Circle neck exercises for the forehead, side of the head, and back of the head. This combination of exercises is called the Travel Around the World sequence. Be sure that you maintain good posture and do not stick your neck out toward your hand. Start with the forehead, side of the head, back of the head, other side of the head, and then reverse the direction. Perform one full set. Follow the Around the World sequence with a neck stretch to release neck tension. The Neck Rotation Pre-Pilates exercise discussed earlier in this section, and the Chest Expansion exercise discussed next, are both good choices.

CHEST EXPANSION

It is a good rule of thumb to follow exercises that strengthen the neck with the Chest Expansion to help release neck tension.

Getting Started

Stand in the appropriate stance for your body, ideally Pilates stance. Stretch your arms forward at shoulder level, shoulder width apart. Take a deep breath in as you press your arms down and slightly behind your hips. Hold your breath for two seconds. On the exhalation, return your arms to shoulder height, reaching forward.

Eventually

Once you have coordinated your breathing with the movement of your arms, add the neck stretch. Starting with the arms extended forward at shoulder level and shoulder width apart, breathe in and press your arms down and slightly behind your hips. Hold your breath as you look over your right shoulder, look center, and then look over your left shoulder. Be sure that you keep your shoulders stationary as you turn your head. To finish, look straight ahead and breathe out as your arms float forward to shoulder level. In the next set, start the neck stretch to the left. Perform 4 sets, alternating the direction of the first neck stretch on each set. **Photos P-T**

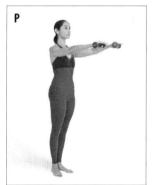 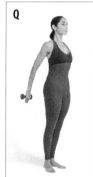 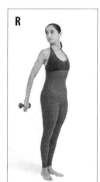 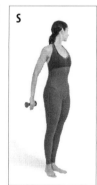 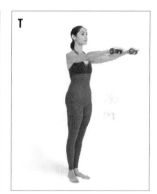

Why It's Beneficial

The Chest Expansion is a breathing exercise that opens the chest, stretches the neck, and strengthens the ocular muscles. It provides a helpful counter stretch when done after any exercise that focuses on strengthening the neck. It is especially beneficial for those who spend a lot of time with computers and mobile devices.

Tips

For students with poor posture, I like to use the cue, "Be the best snob you can be," because it always gets them to open their collarbones wider as the arms reach back.

To help work the ocular muscles, try to see what is behind you as you turn your head over each shoulder.

PRE-PILATES FOR THE JAW

INTRODUCTION

After returning home from our annual staycation one summer, I received an enormous welcome from my furry family members. Before going to bed, I let my dogs out into the backyard for their final potty break of the evening. The last outing in the backyard is generally a quiet one, but on this night things were different. My Great Dane was very excited because he finally had everyone back home, so he began to run circles in the backyard as my Pug/Toy Fox Terrier mix and my Chihuahua chased him. This kind of play usually only happens during the day. It is quite fun to watch them do this, but that night I was distracted, because the Great Dane had just had a bowel movement, and I wanted to pick it up before he stepped in it and made a big mess. It was dark, but we had the security lights on and I had a flashlight, so as the dogs were at the opposite end of the backyard I seized the moment and used my shovel to quickly scoop up the mess. It was then that I discovered what it must feel like to take a punch.

I miscalculated how fast the Great Dane can run and forgot that he often changes direction quickly to throw off his little running mates. I felt his one hundred and forty pounds hit my face at full speed and was certain that my face was broken. With tears running down my face, I looked at myself in the mirror, and I could have sworn that my face was crooked. I applied ice to the right side of my face that night, and spent the next week with a headache and my first black eye, which had to be covered up in a photo shoot for one of my other books. I could barely open my mouth and chewing even the softest foods hurt. After the first few days, I decided to try the Pre-Pilates jaw exercise, with very small range of motion, to try to get my jaw movement back. Little by little, over the course of a month, I regained a full range of movement in my jaw. Before this incident, I had found little reason to do or teach the Pre-Pilates jaw exercise. My experience with jaw pain taught me that this Pre-Pilates exercise can be very beneficial, and my research taught me that it has value for most people.

YAWN/BITE AN APPLE

Getting Started

We all know how contagious yawning can be, but it is also a very good exercise for stretching the jaw, reducing stress, and increasing mental alertness. I will never forget watching the short track speed skating competition during the Winter Olympics one year. One of the sports commentators joked about one of the strongest competitors in the race, thinking that the competitor, who was repeatedly yawning before his race, was showing signs of fatigue. The commentator did not realize that the competitor was doing conscious yawning to give himself a competitive advantage. Yawning creates a state of relaxed alertness and can be a good way to stimulate the part of the brain that affects focus. I did mindful yawning before stepping out onstage as a dancer to reduce performance anxiety, and I always remind my children to do the same before recitals and sports games.

As you sit or stand, bring your attention to activating the muscles in your abdomen, seat, and inner thighs. Look straight ahead, open your mouth wide as you inhale, and exhale as you close your mouth. You will probably start yawning immediately, but it might take a few fake yawns to trigger the real ones. Perform up to 5 times.

Why It's Beneficial

We exercise the jaw joint when we talk and chew food, but it should also be stretched. Opening the mouth wide helps eliminate jaw tension and is a particularly useful exercise for singers, actors, and dancers who want to relax the throat, jaw, face, and body. It is also helpful for people who put tension in their jaws as they grind their teeth, bite their lips, or chew their nails. Jaw exercises can also serve as part of a series of facial exercises to reduce lines and wrinkles in the skin.

Tips
When coordinated with the breath, inhaling and opening the mouth, exhaling and closing the mouth, the jaw exercise brings fresh oxygen into the body's cells. Even the brain may benefit from this exercise, because increased oxygen is said to increase intellectual functioning.

Eventually
After you are comfortable opening your mouth wide in the yawning practice, you might feel comfortable imagining biting into a giant apple. Romana liked to use the image of biting into a Granny Smith apple when giving this jaw-dropping exercise. Sit or stand in your best posture, open your mouth wide and reveal as many teeth as you can. Next, bite down slowly as you focus on the muscles in the front of your neck. Perform 2-4 times. **Photo A**

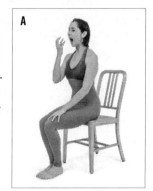

PRE-PILATES FOR THE NOSE

INTRODUCTION
Wiggling the tip of the nose is probably the Pre-Pilates exercise that I use the least. Romana challenged some of her students to wiggle the tip of their nose. In addition to being a party trick, this is an exercise that builds the muscles within the nose. As with wiggling the ears, some of the nose-wiggling muscles have atrophied in humans. But some people can train their nose muscles to move.

WIGGLE THE TIP OF THE NOSE
Getting Started
Sit or stand in front of a mirror. Try to wiggle your nose at varying speeds. **Photo B**

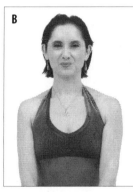

Why It's Beneficial
Wiggling the nose can be part of an exercise routine to shape the nose. Sleeping repeatedly on one side of the face can cause the nose to become crooked, and nose exercises can help. Working the muscles in the nose after nose surgery is important for improving circulation in the facial muscles.

Tips
The Wiggle the Tip of the Nose exercise can also be taught with an emphasis on nasal breathing. My son has allergy-induced asthma and shows considerable improvement when he remembers to keep his mouth closed and breathe through his nose.

Eventually
Flaring the nostrils works the nose muscles in conjunction with nasal breathing. Flare your nostrils on the in-breath and narrow your nostrils on the out-breath. Picture yourself smelling a fresh batch of cookies coming out of the oven on the in-breath. On the out-breath, narrow your nostrils as you pretend that there are stinky socks in the room. Perform 3 sets of breaths.

PRE-PILATES FOR THE EYES

INTRODUCTION

Pilates is a complete system that even addresses the muscles in the eyes. According to his family members, Joe Pilates lost the sight in one of his eyes after a bully threw a stone at his face. Maintaining the vision in his other eye was important to Joe and that is why he created an eye chart to help his students work their extraocular muscles. The extraocular muscles are a group of six muscles that control the movement of the eye, plus one muscle that controls the movement of the eyelid. Many people like to close their eyes when they do Pilates. But it is important to keep the eyes open in order to maintain inner *and* outer awareness. Keeping the eyes focused on the correct spot improves the integrity of the exercise and keeps the Pilates exercises safe. For example, looking at the bellybutton while performing the Hundred is helpful because it keeps the weight of the head toward the powerhouse. Looking at the feet while performing the Hundred is not helpful because it shifts the weight of the head onto the neck and makes the head feel heavier.

The ability to control eye movement can deepen many of the traditional Pilates moves. In exercises that work the waist, like the Criss-Cross and Spine Twist from the Matwork, try to look behind you as you twist. Looking back as you twist helps to deepen your stretch. In exercises like the Neck Roll and Chest Expansion that involve isolating the shoulders while turning the head, isolate your shoulders as you try to see what is behind you.

The ability to control the movement of the eyes can help balance. To improve balance, it is helpful to move the eyes slightly before the head moves. The head is the heaviest part of the body, so moving it without focusing the eyes can throw off the balance. For example, in the advanced version of the Chest Expansion performed on the half toe, I tell students to lead with the eyes when turning the head over one shoulder, and again as the head returns to the center.

It is important not to put unnecessary tension in the eyes while performing Pilates. I frequently have to remind students to relax their eyes. Prolonged exposure to computers, tablets, and mobile phones is the main culprit in eye tension, but stress and lack of sleep play a role as well. When my husband had to go back to Russia for the first time in twenty-four years due to a family emergency, I did my best to take care of my two children and seven pets, while keeping my business running for the entire month of his absence. All went relatively smoothly until two days before his return, when I experienced nearly non-stop twitching in my left eye. This was the first time I had experienced excessive eye twitching and I realized that my body was telling me that stress and insufficient sleep were taking their toll on my body. I did the following Pre-Pilates eye exercises to ease my eye tension and work my eye muscles. By the time my husband returned from Russia, my left eye had stopped twitching.

EYE CIRCLES

Getting Started
Sit or stand with your powerhouse muscles engaged. Draw vertical lines with only your eyes. You can inhale as you move your eyes up, and exhale as you move your eyes down. Next, draw horizontal lines using only your eyes. You can also draw diagonal lines.

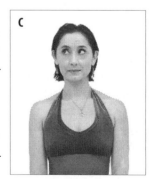

Eventually
Once you are comfortable drawing lines, you can move on to squares, and ultimately finish with your eyes tracing circles. Trace circles going clockwise and then counter-clockwise. **Photo C**

Why It's Beneficial

The Pre-Pilates eye exercises safely relieve digital eye strain and dry eye, and improve concentration. Nearsightedness, farsightedness, and astigmatism are problems with how the eye focuses the light, so some people believe that eye exercises that work on deliberate eye focus can help improve vision and reduce the risk of developing eye diseases. Eye tracking exercises can also be helpful for those who have a lazy eye.

Tips

You can also practice shifting your focus from near to far. Extend your arm out in front of you at eye level with your thumb pointed up. Look at your thumb and then shift your focus farther ahead. Perform 3-5 times.

PRE-PILATES FOR THE EARS

INTRODUCTION

The auricular muscles were once used to move the outer ears to help us hear potential predators, in much the way dogs and cats move their ears. As we evolved, the auricular muscles became nonfunctional in most humans. But a few people still have the ability to move their ears using their auricular muscles.

The Pilates version of wiggling the ears is a scalp exercise that focuses on the occipitals, but it may trigger passive movement in the auricular muscles. Wiggling the ears by moving the scalp will be easier for some than for others, and may have a genetic component. But some believe it can be learned with practice, an example of mind control over the muscles, and potentially Contrology at its best.

WIGGLE EARS

Why It's Beneficial

Romana loved to wiggle her ears with her scalp muscles. The Wiggle the Ears exercise is used for facial toning, especially in the upper face around the eyes, and for hair health and headache relief, as well as entertaining family and friends. The muscles used to wiggle the ears are the occipitals, a group of muscles at the base of the skull. Besides wiggling the ears, they also move the scalp to raise the eyebrows and wrinkle the forehead.

Getting Started

To learn about the occipitals, position your hands near the base of your scalp. A gentle pull on the occipital muscles will produce a subtle movement in the ears.

Eventually

Over time, you may be able to wiggle the ears without the assistance of your fingertips moving the scalp. Remember that the movement is small and almost imperceptible. Perform 5-10 times.

Tips

I noticed that this exercise is easier for me when I am wearing my glasses because the ear movement can be so minute that it is difficult to see. When contracting the occipital muscles while wearing glasses, you can feel a slight movement in the eyeglass frames as they move on the bridge of your nose. Pull the lenses of your glasses closer to your eyes as you contract your occipital muscles. You will naturally pull your ears back as you pull your glasses back on your nose. **Photo D**

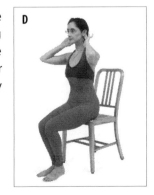

WORKS CITED

Biel, Andrew. *Trail Guide to the Body: How to Locate Muscles, Bones and More.* Consolidated Press, 1997.

Carr, Coeli. "Still Swinging." *TIME*, 19 July 2004, www.time.com/time/generations/ article/0,9171,1101040719-662789,00.html. Accessed 21 Nov. 2004.

Gallagher, Sean, and Romana Kryzanowska. *The Joseph H. Pilates Archive Collection.* Trans-Atlantic Publications Inc., 2000.

Ray, Marie Beynon. "Cutting a Fine Figure." *Collier's, The National Weekly,* 18 August 1934, pp. 21 & 30.

Wake-Up Exercises

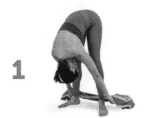

1

p. 64   CAROLA'S STRETCH

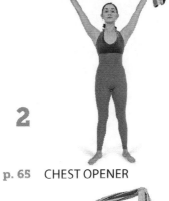

2

p. 65   CHEST OPENER

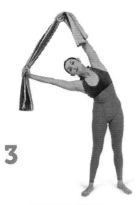

3

p. 65   SIDE TO SIDE

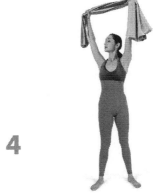

4

p. 66   TWIST, REACH, AROUND THE WORLD

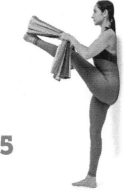

5

p. 67   TREE STANDING

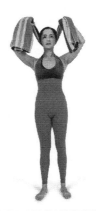

6

p. 68   ASSISTED NECK STRETCH

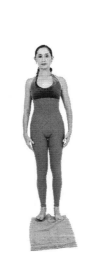

7

p. 69   TOWEL FOOTWORK STANDING

WAKE-UP EXERCISES

INTRODUCTION

In addition to film footage of Joe teaching and demonstrating his Method, we also have a film (in which he wears swim trunks) about how to work the body while taking a shower and toweling off *(Archival Footage of Joseph Pilates)*. In the film, he shows how an ordinary morning routine can be a full body workout which improves stretch, strength, and balance control. Joe frequently advised his students to take an invigorating shower in the morning and also encouraged them to perform Wake-Up Exercises with a towel after the shower. Romana said that Joe liked to give these exercises to people who travel for business, because they can be done in a small space, like a hotel bathroom. Many of the Wake-Up Exercises are done with the arms raised, so be sure to rest your arms down by your sides between exercises.

You have the option of doing the full routine in the order described in this chapter, or you can focus on one or two of the Wake-Up Exercises before going into your Matwork routine.

CAROLA'S STRETCH

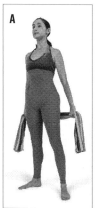
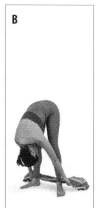

Getting Started
Stand with your feet slightly apart and hold a rolled bath towel behind you, below hip level. Your arms reach toward the floor and your hands are shoulder width apart on the towel, palms facing away from you **(Photo A)**. Take a deep breath, bring your chin toward your chest, and breathe out as you slide the towel down the backs of your legs **(Photo B)**. While the ultimate goal is to roll down with straight legs, it is perfectly acceptable to soften the backs of the knees. Next, lift your C-curve as you breathe in, and roll up your spine. Perform up to 3 times.

Eventually
The final version of this exercise includes a stretch in the chest and shoulders. After you roll the towel down the backs of your legs, lift your arms above your head while remaining in forward flexion **(Photo C)**. Remember to move deliberately. Make sure that you do not exceed your safe range of movement on the stretch. To finish, lower your arms toward your heels and roll up to standing with your arms long, behind your legs. Perform up to 3 times.

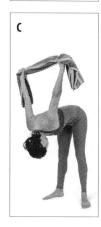

Why It's Beneficial
Joe Pilates' student, Carola Strauss Trier, described this exercise as "Towel Trick 1" in her Pilates book for children (Trier 38). It is similar to the Peel Down from the Wall Series, the Roll-Up from the Matwork, the Reverse Push Through on the Cadillac, and the Round Back/Hug from the Short Box Series on the Reformer. Carola's Stretch opens the low back, chest, and shoulders, and also works the breathing, develops articulation in the spine, and stretches the hamstrings.

Tips
Some people are distracted by the stretch in the backs of the legs and forget to let the head hang as they bend forward over their legs. Remember to relax your neck as you go into forward flexion at the start of this exercise.

CHEST OPENER

Getting Started
Stand with your feet slightly apart. You can work up to performing the movement with your feet together. Hold a rolled bath towel with your arms in front of your thighs (**Photo D**). As you extend your arms forward and up, remember to keep your powerhouse muscles engaged so as not to arch your back. Lift your arms to the point at which your posture remains unaffected by the movement (**Photo E**). After lifting your arms, lower them back down in front of your legs. Perform 3 arm raises.

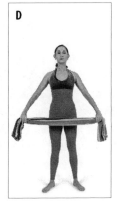 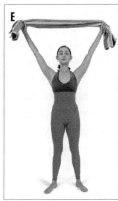

Why It's Beneficial
The Chest Opener exercise increases shoulder flexibility, stretches the chest muscles, and develops powerhouse control as the arms move. This is a good exercise for people who spend a lot of time hunched over a computer. This exercise is similar to the Flat Back exercise from the Short Box Series on the Reformer. Both exercises focus on lifting the sternum and lengthening the spine.

Tips
The Chest Opener exercise is meant for people with healthy shoulders. Although the goal of this exercise is to get the hands shoulder width apart on the towel, it should be introduced with the hands placed wider than shoulder width on a long bath towel. Observe your form and anticipate when you have reached your safe limit.

Eventually
If you are able to maintain good posture on the first part of the Chest Opener exercise, you can attempt to take your arms behind you after you extend your arms forward and up. Be sure that you keep your arms stretched and your shoulders even. Imagine that your shoulder blades are slippery bars of soap, sliding down your back as you move your arms. Repeat the movement from back to front. If you maintain control through your shoulders and are able to isolate your torso from the movement in your arms, you can move your hands closer to shoulder width apart on the towel. Perform up to 3 sets. **Photos F-G**

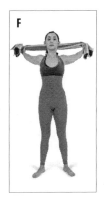 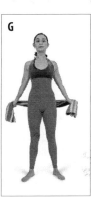

SIDE TO SIDE

Getting Started
Before practicing Side to Side standing, practice the Side to Side exercise sitting on the front edge of a chair. After placing your hands shoulder width apart on a rolled towel, raise your arms to frame your face. Keep your gaze straight ahead as you bend from side to side. It's not easy to recognize unevenness in the hips while performing a side bend in a standing posture, but when one hip lifts off the seat of a chair while sitting, it is more noticeable.

Why It's Beneficial
The Side to Side exercise stretches and strengthens the sides of the torso. It is similar to the Side To Side exercise from the Short Box Series on the Reformer.

Tips
It can be a challenge to keep the arms equidistant from the ears as the torso and arms reach to one side. Consider omitting the rolled towel initially. Extend your arms up and interlace your thumbs as you bend from side to side.

Eventually

Stand with your feet slightly apart and your powerhouse lifted. After placing your hands shoulder width apart on a rolled towel, raise your arms, keeping them in your field of vision. With your arms equidistant from your ears, bend to one side for a count of three, and return to center for a count of three. Keep your weight equal on both feet throughout the movement, and keep your gaze straight ahead without letting your arms cross in front of your face. Perform 2 sets. **Photos H-J**

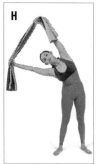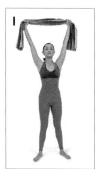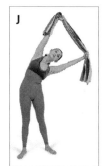

TWIST, REACH, AND AROUND THE WORLD

Getting Started

Do the Twist and the Reach as an introduction to the Around the World exercise.

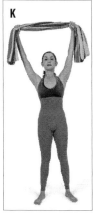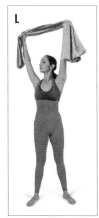

Twist: Stand with your feet slightly apart and hold a rolled towel in front of your thighs. With your hands positioned shoulder width apart on the towel, raise your arms to frame your face. Lift through your waistline and twist tall without moving your hips. Be sure to emphasize the out-breath as you twist. On the in-breath your torso returns to the front of the room. Repeat to the other side. **Photos K-L**

Reach: For an added challenge, you can combine the Twist from the waist with a reach bending forward. Romana used to teach this exercise as a precursor to the advanced Standing Twist at the end of the Matwork. (The advanced Standing Twist involves pivoting on the half toes, rotating from the waist, and bending forward while reaching for the back ankle.)

To perform the Reach exercise, stand with your feet slightly apart, powerhouse engaged, and your hands positioned shoulder width apart on the towel. Raise your arms to frame your face. Moving from your waist and not your hips, rotate your torso to the right, bend over your right leg and remain in forward flexion as you center your torso on the midline, so that your ears are between your legs. Then, rotate your waist to the left, so that you are bent over your left leg. Lift your powerhouse and roll up your spine with your arms reaching toward the ceiling and your torso still facing the left front corner of the room. Bring your torso back to center and repeat the sequence with your waist rotating to the left. To deepen your hamstring stretch, try to "kiss each knee" as you bend over each leg. Perform 4 times. **Photos M-R**

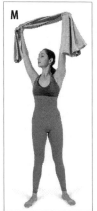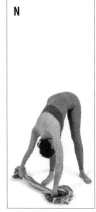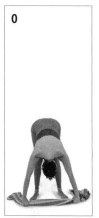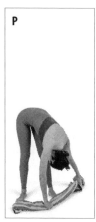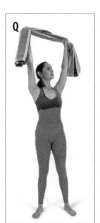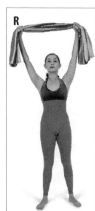

Tips

Imagine that your torso is a wet towel being wrung dry as you twist from your waistline. Remember to isolate your hips from the twist in your waist and upper back.

Eventually

Around the World: For the ultimate challenge, perform Around the World. Stand with your feet slightly apart and hold the towel over your head. Perform a side bend to the right **(Photo S)**, and fold your torso over your right leg with your nose to your right knee **(Photo T)**, hips always facing forward. Stay folded over as you center your torso on the midline and bring your head between your legs **(Photo U)**. From the stretch down the midline, fold over your left leg **(Photo V)**. Then rotate from your waist so that your chest faces the front of the room, your arms reaching to the left in a side bend **(Photo W)**, then returning upright to center **(Photo X)**. Repeat the movement starting to the left and coming up on the right. Perform 4 times.

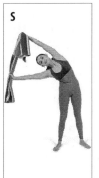 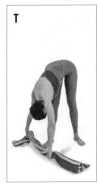 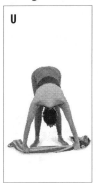 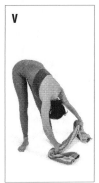 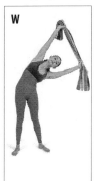 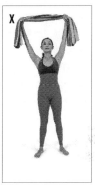

Why It's Beneficial

The Twist, Reach, and Around the World exercises stretch and strengthen the sides of the torso, work the waistline, stretch the hamstrings, and invigorate the whole body. They are standing versions of the Twist, Reach, and Around the World from the Short Box Series on the Reformer.

TREE STANDING

Getting Started

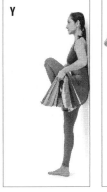

Learn the Tree Standing exercise standing against a wall. With your feet slightly in front of the wall, press your hips, back, and shoulders against the wall while holding a folded towel in both hands. Your hands should be at least shoulder width apart on the towel. Next, lift your knee to your chest and place the sole of your foot on the towel. Without lifting your shoulders, bend your arms as you pull up on the towel and draw your knee closer to your chest **(Photo Y)**. To stretch your hamstring, extend the lower half of your leg upward, still holding the towel **(Photo Z)**. Try to keep your knee to your chest with your shoulders pressing back into the wall as your leg extends. Straightening the leg is not as important as keeping the thigh close to the chest. Perform 3 times and repeat to the other side.

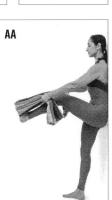

Tips

The towel can be used to promote circulation in the bottom of the foot. Before starting the Tree Standing, lean against the wall, holding the towel. Lift your knee and place the sole of your foot on the towel. To massage the foot, vigorously slide the towel from side to side so that it rubs the pressure points on the bottom of your foot. If possible, try to stretch your leg forward while rubbing the towel against the bottom of your foot. Perform 1 time on each leg. **Photo AA**

Why It's Beneficial

The Tree Standing exercise stretches the back, hamstrings, and Achilles tendons, and helps balance control. It resembles the Tree from the Short Box Series on the Reformer.

Eventually

To develop better balance, do the Tree Standing without leaning on a wall. **Photos BB-CC**

ASSISTED NECK STRETCH

Getting Started

Stand in a comfortable stance with your powerhouse lifted and your hands holding a rolled towel, which is draped around the base of your skull. Lift the ends of the towel forward and up, slightly above your eye level. Create gentle traction as you lengthen the back of your neck **(Photo DD)**. Next, hold the ends of the towel out at your eye level as you bend your head forward while applying a very gentle pressure on the towel **(Photo EE)**. Then lift your face slightly and press the back of your head into the towel, while pulling the ends of the towel forward and up to provide support **(Photo FF)**. As you lengthen the back of your neck and push your head back into the towel, imagine that your towel is a hammock giving your head a place to rest. To continue the stretches, gently tilt your head so that one ear moves toward your shoulder while pulling carefully forward and up on the towel with the top arm **(Photo GG)**. Repeat on the other side. Perform 1 set front and back, and 1 set side-to-side.

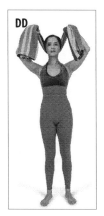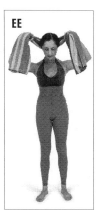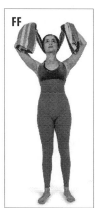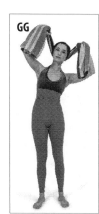

Why It's Beneficial

The Assisted Neck Stretch promotes circulation in the neck, and the towel provides additional stretch, support, and gentle traction.

Tips

This exercise comes toward the end of the Wake-Up Exercise sequence because it is best to stretch the neck when the body is warmed up. Before starting the exercise, place the rolled towel behind your neck and gently slide the towel from side to side to increase circulation in your neck.

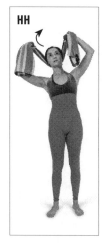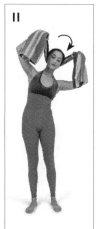

The arms are active in the Assisted Neck Stretch because they are supporting the heaviest part of the body. It may be necessary to let the arms rest long by the sides of the body from time to time during the exercise.

Eventually

In time, you can add slow neck rolls while gently pulling the ends of the towel out at eye level. Your shoulders move *a little* as your head and neck move. Perform 1-2 neck rolls in each direction. **Photos HH-II**

TOWEL FOOTWORK STANDING

Getting Started
Performing Towel Footwork in a standing posture is an extra challenge because of the added body weight in the legs. It is best to learn this exercise in a seated position. The Towel Footwork performed in a seated position is described on page 14, in the feet section of the Pre-Pilates chapter. **Photo JJ**

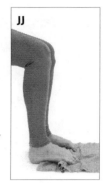

Why It's Beneficial
In Pilates, the arch is considered the powerhouse of the foot. This exercise is designed to keep the arches lifted. Because many people wear closed toed shoes so much of the time, exercises like this one are a good remedy for stiff, sore feet.

Eventually
Stand at one end of the towel with your feet and legs parallel and apart. Your bellybutton is lifting, your seat muscles are activated, and your inner thighs are hugging the midline. One foot and then the other pulls the towel toward you, much like the paws of a cat kneading a blanket. Reversing the movement is especially hard in the standing posture. Imagine that you are digging your toes into sand as you try to push the towel away from you with one foot at a time. Perform once in each direction. **Photo KK**

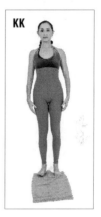

Tips
Be sure that you engage your seat in order to align your feet. Keeping the buttocks muscles engaged helps maintain the lift in both the outer and inner blades of the feet as they go into the dome shape. As you make the dome shape with your feet, imagine that your feet are eating up the towel.

WORKS CITED

Archival Footage of Joseph Pilates. Historical film footage compiled and edited by Power Pilates, 2005.

Trier, Carola S. *Exercise: What It Is, What It Does*. Greenwillow Books, 1982.

Basic Matwork with a Towel Pre-Pilates and Beyond

Basic Matwork with a Towel

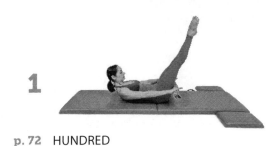

1 p. 72   HUNDRED

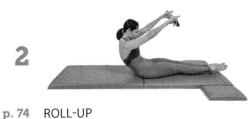

2 p. 74   ROLL-UP

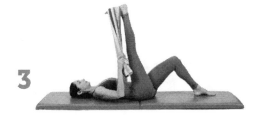

3 p. 75   HAMSTRING STRETCH
       p. 76   SINGLE LEG CIRCLES

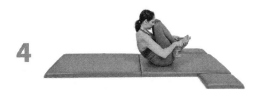

4 p. 77   ROLLING LIKE A BALL

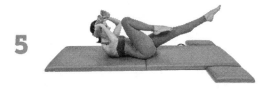

5 p. 78   SINGLE LEG STRETCH

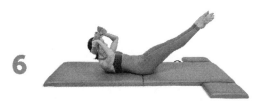

6 p. 79   DOUBLE LEG STRETCH

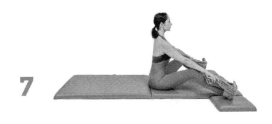

7 p. 80   SPINE STRETCH FORWARD

BASIC MATWORK WITH A TOWEL

INTRODUCTION

The Short Pole and the Magic Circle are common additions to the Matwork in the studio, but a rolled towel can work just as well. Using a rolled towel as you do your Matwork can help you check your upper body alignment when it is held taut between your hands, can deepen the stretch in your leg when it is wrapped around your foot, and can provide neck support when it is held at the base of your skull. A standard size hand towel works best for all exercises with the exception of the Hamstring Stretch, which works better for most people when performed with a bath towel.

The Basic Matwork routine is meant to be done in a specific order. For each of the Matwork exercises in this chapter, you have three options to choose from. There is an introductory variation described in the *Getting Started* section, a deeper practice variation described in the *Eventually* section, and for added variety, there is the variation done with a rolled towel. If neither of the three options is a good fit for you, skip the exercise and move on to the next exercise in the sequence that is suitable for you.

HUNDRED

Getting Started

Lying on the mat, place a few folded hand towels under your head. The towels will help you stay in your powerhouse by gently bringing the weight of your head toward your center. The folded towels also help avoid neck strain. To help support your back, rest your feet on the mat with your legs bent at about ninety degrees.

It is best to concentrate on only one or two components of the Hundred when first learning it. A good way to break down the Hundred is to start with the breathing on its own, next do the arm pumping on its own, and then put the two components together. This progression can be spread out over the course of a few workouts.

Breathe in for five counts and breathe out for five counts. Remember to breathe through your nose to avoid shallow breaths. If you are breathing well, challenge yourself with a longer exhalation. Breathe in for four counts and breathe out for six counts to stay within the frame of ten counts. There is no need to do the full ten sets. Two or three sets of mindful breathing with correct body placement are enough. The focus should be on quality breathing and getting the last drop of air out through the nose before taking the next breath.

After you are comfortable with breathing to counts, add the arm pumping motion. As you pump your arms vigorously, six to eight inches above the mat, imagine that you are dribbling two basketballs that are placed an arm's length away. When the time is right, combine the breathing and the arm movement.

Once the breathing sequence and the arm movement are coordinated, you can lift your head off the mat. This is an all or nothing position. Either your head is all the way down on the folded towels, or it is all the way up where you can see your bellybutton, while still maintaining a small space between your chin and your chest. The base of your shoulder blades should touch the mat while the back of your head and the top of your shoulders peel away from the mat. Start with 3-5 sets, and over time, work up to the full 10 sets. If necessary, you can alternate the position of your head during the exercise. I like to use the following pattern when students are first learning to perform the full 10 sets: head up for three sets, head down for four sets, head up for the final three sets.

Why It's Beneficial

The Hundred is a very challenging exercise with many components. The pumping motion of the arms helps circulate the blood and gets the body warmed up for the rest of the workout. The breathing improves the stamina and oxygenates the blood. Raising the legs and/or head above the mat deepens the powerhouse strength.

I have noticed that the Hundred is more challenging for me now than it was when I was a Pilates apprentice twenty years ago. My improved understanding of the nuances of the Hundred, plus the fact that I am more honest with myself about where the working height of my legs should be, has made it a much harder exercise than it once was. Romana often said, "I hate the Hundred and I never do it!" I used to think she was joking, but maybe there was some truth to what she said. The Hundred is challenging, but it is an integral part of the Pilates Method, and can be modified in multiple ways to accommodate all students.

Tips

From a Pilates point of view, the neck is considered the second powerhouse. It is best not to lift your head off the mat until you are more familiar with the other components of the Hundred. The heaviest part of the body is the head. Because of its weight, lifting your head before you are ready can be very dangerous.

Eventually

When you have developed a reasonable amount of powerhouse strength and coordination, it's time to add the legs. For safety, start with your knees to your chest in order to help keep your back anchored to the mat.

For more of a challenge, move your legs into a tabletop shape with your knees bent at ninety degrees (**Photo A**). Eventually, stretch your legs long while rotating them into Pilates stance (**Photo B**). Your legs should be placed high enough to avoid arching your back.

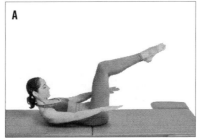
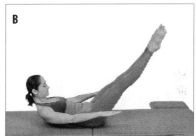

HUNDRED WITH A TOWEL

The Hundred performed with the Short Pole inspired these variations.

Start with the knees bent at ninety degrees, with the towel under the lifted legs and hands shoulder width apart on the towel. Keep the towel taut as you pump (**Photo C**). When you have developed more powerhouse strength, stretch your legs long while rotating them into Pilates stance (**Photo D**). Pumping the arms with the towel under the legs will help you feel how to peel the head, neck, and tops of the shoulders off the mat.

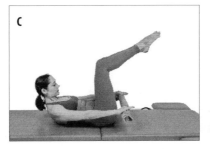
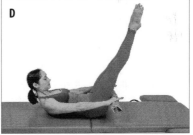

Eventually, you can pump the arms while holding the towel taut above your lifted legs (**Photo E**). This variation forces the working height of the legs to go closer to the mat, deepening the work in the powerhouse. If your powerhouse is strong enough, there should be no strain in the low back in this variation of the Hundred with the towel.

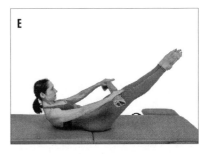

ROLL-UP

Getting Started

You should be able to do the Roll Down with ease before you attempt the Roll-Up. To do the Roll Down, sit with your legs bent and your feet hooked under a low piece of furniture. Your feet can be together or parallel and apart. I prefer feet together because it is easier to find the midline and access the inner thigh muscles with the legs together. Place your hands lightly on the back of each thigh, just above the backs of the knees, and go into a C-curve with your waistline lifted and your head curled forward into your powerhouse. Avoiding a white-knuckle grip, pull your bellybutton back toward the mat as your hands remain on the same spot behind your thighs. Before your arms straighten completely, roll forward to the starting position.

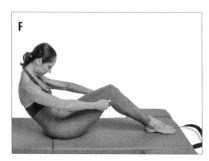

Once you understand how to roll through your spine in a small range of motion, you can continue to roll your spine back into the mat beyond the point of straightening your arms. After rolling back to the point where your arms are straight, slide your hands down the back of each thigh as you roll deeper into the mat. If you can increase your range of movement without using your hands to roll back up, you can perform the Roll Down with the full range of movement. Eventually, you can take your feet out from under the low piece of furniture. Remember that your head is the last part of the body to reach onto the mat and the first part of the body to come up off the mat. Perform 3-5 repetitions. **Photo F**

Eventually

Once you have mastered the Roll Down, you can work on the Roll-Up. Begin lying face up with your legs long and feet together. Your arms reach toward the ceiling at a ninety-degree angle to the mat. Lift the back of your head off the mat and peel your spine away from the mat as you bend forward. You can soften your knees and hold the backs of your legs as you sit up. To keep tension out of your neck, remember to let your head hang as you bend forward.

When you can do the Roll-Up without putting your hands behind your thighs as you sit up, you can try to keep your arms at a ninety-degree angle to your shoulders as you peel off the mat and roll back onto it. To begin, extend your arms overhead and back toward the mat. Your arms do not touch the mat. Be aware of the natural tendency to arch your back as the arms move back toward your ears. Engage your abdominals to avoid arching your back. *Your arms should only move at the beginning of the Roll-Up, from home position toward the ceiling* (**Photos H-I**), *and at the end of the Roll-Up, from reaching toward the ceiling to home position.* This means that your arms only move when your head is on the mat. Your arms should always be at a ninety-degree angle to your shoulders as you peel your body away from the mat and roll your back onto the mat.

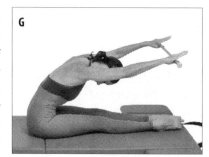

It is important to squeeze the seat muscles and press the backs of the inner thighs together so that the heels stay glued together and the back does not strain. As you roll up, imagine that your spine is a piece of masking tape being peeled slowly off the mat. As you reach toward your toes, be sure that you keep your arms at shoulder level (**Photo G**). When you are ready to roll back onto the mat, focus on curling forward to work your abdominals more deeply. To provide a nice feeling of opposition, you can float the crown of your head forward as you pull your waist back. Perform 3-5 times.

Why It's Beneficial

The Roll-Up works the articulation of the spine and strengthens the powerhouse muscles on a more challenging level than the introductory Roll Down. Joe Pilates believed that a person is as young as their spine is healthy. To keep the spine healthy, he created exercises like the Roll-Up.

Tips

Remember not to perform a "karate chop" with your arms in order to sit up. Try to sit up using your muscle strength instead of using momentum in your arms. You are learning Pilates, not "karate-lates!"

The Roll-Up can shine a light on muscle imbalances. Observe your movement as you peel off the mat and check to see if you are favoring one side. If you lean to one side as you sit up, that might be a sign that you are relying on the stronger side of your torso to sit up.

ROLL-UP WITH THE TOWEL

The Roll-Up performed with the Short Pole inspired this variation of the Roll-Up.

Put your hands shoulder width apart on the towel, lie on your back, and raise your arms toward the ceiling. If you are able to keep your back on the mat, extend your arms back toward your ears. Keep the towel taut as you roll up and roll down. **Photos H-L**

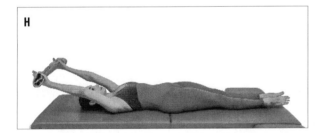
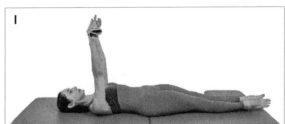
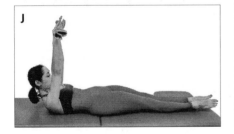
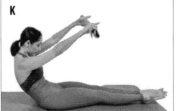
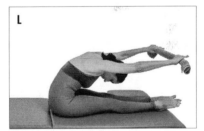

HAMSTRING STRETCH

Getting Started

Lie on the mat with your legs bent at roughly ninety degrees, feet resting on the mat. You can put a few folded hand towels under your head, if you need help lengthening the back of your neck. With one foot resting on the mat, extend your other leg toward the ceiling. Keeping the bottom leg bent makes it easier to keep your hips anchored while stretching your working leg. When your raised leg is in Pilates stance, you should be able to see the inside of your ankle bone. With your arms long by your sides, focus on pulling your bellybutton deeper into the mat as you lengthen the back of your working knee a little more. **Photo M**

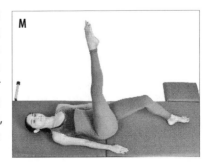

Tips
Never hold your stretches longer than three seconds. No matter how flexible you are, muscles held in a stretch for longer than three seconds tend to trigger a protective reflex, in which the muscle you are trying to lengthen begins to contract.

Eventually
You can stack your hands behind your thigh and repeat the stretch with the assistance of your hands. Do not interlace your fingers, because interlaced fingers can put tension in the shoulders and neck. Avoid putting your hands behind your knee because that increases the likelihood of bending the leg during the hamstring stretch. Gently pull your leg up toward the ceiling as your bellybutton sinks down into the mat for a three second stretch. Emphasize the length of your leg and not the height of the leg.

Why It's Beneficial
The Hamstring Stretch often precedes the Single Leg Circles in the Matwork series. It is a safe way to limber the back of the leg because the back has support.

HAMSTRING STRETCH WITH THE TOWEL
The Hamstring Stretch with the Magic Circle is the inspiration for this Hamstring Stretch with the Towel.

Lie on your back with one leg bent at ninety degrees, foot resting on the mat. Bend your other leg toward your chest and put a rolled bath towel on the sole of your foot. Create two opposing lines of energy as you stretch the working leg toward the ceiling while pressing your working hip down into the mat.

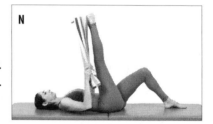

If you are ready for a deeper stretch, bend your arms as you pull on the towel, without bending your raised leg **(Photo N)**. After holding the stretch with bent arms for three counts, reduce the intensity of the stretch in the raised leg by stretching your arms and letting your leg go a little lower. Perform 1-3 times on each leg, for no more than three seconds at a time. You can follow the Hamstring Stretch on each leg with the Single Leg Circles. See the next exercise for details.

SINGLE LEG CIRCLES
Getting Started
After limbering the back of your leg with the Hamstring Stretch described earlier, go into the Single Leg Circles. Keeping your supporting leg bent makes it easier to keep your hips anchored as you stretch your working leg. Remember to rotate your raised leg in Pilates stance to avoid gripping your hip flexor and/or overworking the top of the thigh.

With your working leg raised and in line with your midline, initiate the first set of leg circles with your leg crossing over your midline at the *top* of the circle, and opening no farther than the shoulder width to come back up to home position. On the second set of leg circles, your leg moves from the midline toward the outside shoulder and crosses over the midline at the *bottom* of the circle, on its way back up to home position. Make sure that both of your hips remain on the mat as your leg circles.

Keep the circles small in order to keep the focus on the stability of the torso. Increase the circumference of the circles only if the torso is able to remain isolated from the leg movement. Circle the leg across the body 5 times and reverse. Repeat on the other side.

Why It's Beneficial
The Single Leg Circles strengthen the sides of the torso and work the leg in the hip socket.

Tips
Use imagery to enhance your movement:

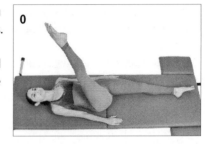

Imagine that you have a hot cup of coffee on your bellybutton as you circle your leg. To avoid spills, keep your torso stable as your top leg moves.

Imagine your top leg is a paintbrush. Your foot should remain long and loose like the soft bristles of the brush while your leg remains straight like the long handle. Imagine painting each circle a different color.

Eventually
As your torso strength and leg flexibility improve, move your supporting foot forward on the mat, eventually stretching your supporting leg long on the mat **(Photo 0)**. Circle the working leg across the body 5 times and reverse. Repeat on the other side.

TOWEL UNDER THE THIGH

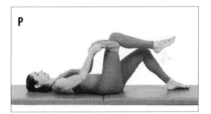

If your hip is delicate, you can support the circling leg with a towel under your thigh and keep your leg bent as your arms move the thigh in a circular motion. See page 25 in the Hip section of the Pre-Pilates chapter for details. **Photo P**

ROLLING LIKE A BALL

Getting Started

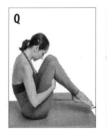
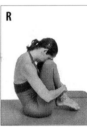

Sit on the mat with your legs bent to your chest and your feet close to your seat. You can hold the backs of your thighs **(Photo Q)**, and if your knees are healthy, work up to holding your ankles for a deeper stretch **(Photo R)**. Your knees are slightly open with your heels together. Your head floats toward your knees as you pull up in your low back and lift through your waistline. Once in position, balance on your tailbone with your feet hovering above the mat. The more compact you get, the more challenging it is to hold your balance.

Eventually
As your powerhouse strength increases and your balance improves, you can start rolling. Initiate the rolling action from your abdominals while keeping your gaze toward your bellybutton. Roll back to your shoulders as your bottom and waist lift away from the mat. <u>Do not let your head or neck touch the mat as you roll back.</u> Attempt to roll up to sitting without letting your feet touch the mat.

Remember that maintaining good form is more important than returning all the way to the seated position. It is all right to feel like a turtle that is stuck on its back. A small range of rolling movement with the head, knees, and feet tucked is better than using momentum from the feet and/or knees to perform the full range of movement. Perform 6 times.

NOTE: People with scoliosis and/or delicate backs should not roll. Instead, focus on the balance only.

Balancing in a ball shape develops balance control and powerhouse strength. Rolling Like a Ball massages the pressure points along both sides of the spine, and also improves balance control and powerhouse strength. Rolling Like a Ball is the foundation for other exercises from the Matwork like Open Leg Rocker and Teaser.

Tips

Romana liked to say, "Pretend your head is a block of wood that is being held in a vice" to get her student to bring his head between his knees in the ball shape.

You will probably lift your shoulders in your effort to balance, so remember to let your shoulders "melt" and redirect your energy to pulling your bellybutton in and up.

Rolling should never be performed on hard flooring without a mat.

ROLLING LIKE A BALL WITH A TOWEL

This variation of Rolling Like a Ball can help you keep your heels close to your seat in the ball shape. Balance with the towel under your feet as you bend your elbows and keep your shoulders down. Once you have a strong balance in the ball shape, you can try rolling. **Photos S-U**

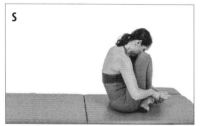
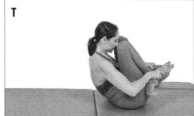
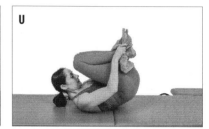

SINGLE LEG STRETCH

Getting Started

Lie on the mat with a few folded hand towels under your head and your feet resting on the mat. Next, bend one leg and hug the back of the thigh to your chest. Your hands are stacked but not interlaced and your thumbs remain with your fingers, instead of being used for gripping. Your elbows lift away from the mat as your bellybutton sinks into the mat. Next, extend your other leg toward the ceiling while rotating it into a Pilates stance. Keeping the bent leg parallel, and the extended leg in Pilates stance develops concentration and coordination. Alternate hugging one leg at a time. Once you have the coordination of the movement in your limbs, you can try a few sets with your head raised off the mat and your extended leg slightly lower than it was when your head was resting on the mat. **Photo V**

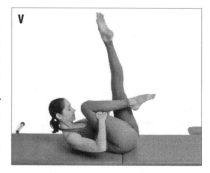

Why It's Beneficial

The Single Leg Stretch strengthens the abdominal muscles and stretches the back. It also works the backs of the arms.

Tips

Remember that the reason you pull the bent leg into your chest is to stretch out your back. Pointing your elbows to the sides of the room as you hug each leg strengthens the backs of your arms and opens your back, while closing your rib cage. When you know why you are doing a movement, you will do it more carefully.

Eventually

If you have healthy knees, hug one leg to your chest with both hands stacked on your shin. Over time you may be able to progress to swapping the hand positions on the bent leg, placing the outside hand on the ankle, and the inside hand on the shin. This improves the alignment of the hip, knee, and ankle of the bent leg, deepens the stretch in the back, and works the coordination. Alternate hugging each leg while extending the other leg in front of you **(Photo W)**. Using the image of a bow and arrow, imagine that you are pulling the notched arrow back on the string of a bow as you pull your knee to your chest. When you release your bent leg, watch the arrow travel in slow motion as your leg extends in front of you, toward your target. Perform 3-5 sets.

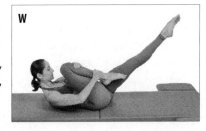

SINGLE LEG STRETCH WITH A TOWEL

This variation of Single Leg Stretch offers extra neck support. It helps you focus on your powerhouse muscles as you alternate stretching one leg in Pilates stance with your heel in line with your midline, while bending the other leg to your chest. As you do this, place the hand towel under the base of your skull and pull forward very gently, holding the ends of the towel out at your eye level. **Photos X-Y**

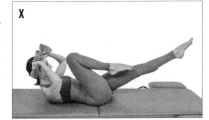
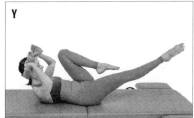

DOUBLE LEG STRETCH

Getting Started

Lie on the mat with a few folded hand towels under your head and your knees bent into your chest. As in the Rolling Like a Ball position, your knees are slightly apart and your heels are together. Place your hands behind your thighs for a gentle stretch. If you have healthy knees, grab your ankles for a more intense stretch in the back. If you are ready to lift your head off the mat, remember to keep your gaze consistently on your bellybutton and to keep the movement of your limbs within your field of vision. With your heels remaining together, stretch your arms and legs toward the ceiling. Inhale as you stretch out long and thin **(Photo Z)**, and exhale as your knees and arms come back to starting position **(Photo BB)**. As you stretch your arms and legs, imagine that you are opening like the petals of a blooming flower. When you come back into starting position, imagine that you are closing like a clamshell. Perform 3-5 times.

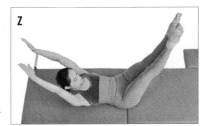

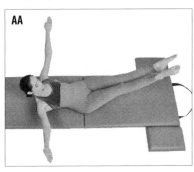

Why It's Beneficial

The Double Leg Stretch is a more intense version of the Single Leg Stretch. It works coordination of the breath with the movement in the limbs. The Double Leg Stretch strengthens the stomach when the legs extend and stretches the back when the knees bend into the chest.

Eventually

As you gain more powerhouse strength and coordination, you may be able to progress to the full arm movement. After the arms and legs extend **(Photo Z)**, hold the legs steady as your arms open to a T-shape **(Photo AA)**. Return to home position with the knees to the chest to finish **(Photo BB)**. Perform 3-5 times.

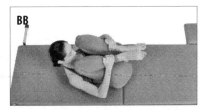

Tips

If your arms go too far behind you during the stretch, you will probably change your head position. Remember that the heaviest part of your body is your head, and that is why it is crucial that your head move toward your center as your limbs extend away from your center. Extending the arms and legs toward the ceiling will help you focus on your powerhouse strength.

DOUBLE LEG STRETCH WITH A TOWEL

This variation of the Double Leg Stretch offers extra neck support to allow more focus on the powerhouse muscles as you stretch both legs forward and hold for the count of three, and bend both knees to your chest. Place the hand towel under the base of your skull and pull forward and up very gently, holding the ends of the towel at eye level. **Photos CC-DD**

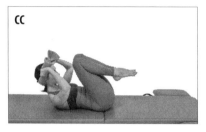
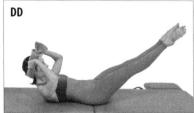

SPINE STRETCH FORWARD

Getting Started

Sit tall with your legs slightly wider than the mat. If you can't sit with your back straight, bend your knees slightly. Knees and toes point to the ceiling and the middle of the knees are aligned over the second toes. To keep your feet flexed, imagine that your feet are slices of toast coming out of the slots of a toaster oven. There is a connection between your feet and your seat. The more you push out of your heels, the more you will activate your seat. However, if the stretch in the hamstrings is too intense, it is best to keep the feet long and loose.

Lift your powerhouse and maintain the lift in your sides as you put your fingertips on the mat in front of you and lower your head. While breathing out, slide your fingertips forward on the mat while pulling your waist back. Focus on emptying your lungs as you bend your torso forward. To avoid collapsing in the waistline, imagine that you are lifting your waist over a small picket fence as you bend forward.

Why It's Beneficial

The Spine Stretch Forward opens the low back, stretches the backs of the legs, and helps empty the lungs.

Eventually

If your shoulders are healthy and you can keep tension out of them, lift your arms in front of you at shoulder height. If you can keep your back lifted, straighten your legs in the narrow straddle position. Lift tall on your in-breath and imagine that your arms are sliding forward, across a table as you bury the crown of your head toward your bellybutton while breathing out and bending forward **(Photo EE)**. When you have no more air left to breathe out, inhale as you roll up your spine, sitting tall. Perform 3 times.

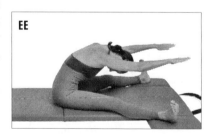

SPINE STRETCH FORWARD WITH TOWELS

To deepen the stretch in both the back and the hamstrings, Romana used to have us reach for our insteps with bent legs and try to keep our grip on them as we stretched our legs. The Spine Stretch Forward with the hands on the insteps is the inspiration for this variation of the Spine Stretch Forward using towels.

Wrap a hand towel around each foot to facilitate the stretch. With your hands on both ends of each towel, soften your knees and sit tall with your legs in a small straddle, feet flexed **(Photo FF)**. After taking a deep breath, bend forward at your waist, empty your lungs, and slide your feet forward in a V-shape as your arms stretch. For an even deeper stretch, you can keep your elbows bent as you slide your legs out in the V-shape **(Photo GG)**.

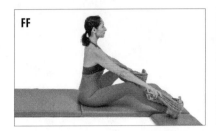 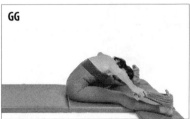

Joe's Archival Routine

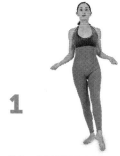

1

p. 84   JUMPING ROPE

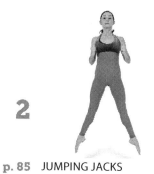

2

p. 85   JUMPING JACKS

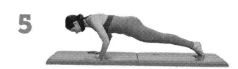

3

p. 86   ROLL-UP

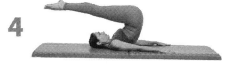

4

p. 86   ROLL OVER

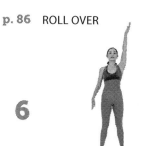

5

p. 87   PUSH-UPS

6

p. 87   SAW STANDING

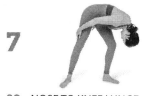

7

p. 88   NOSE TO KNEE LUNGE

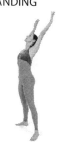

8

p. 88   ARM SWINGING BACKBEND

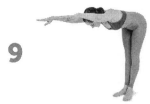

9

p. 89   HUGGING THE SUN

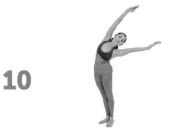

10

p. 90   ORBITING THE SUN

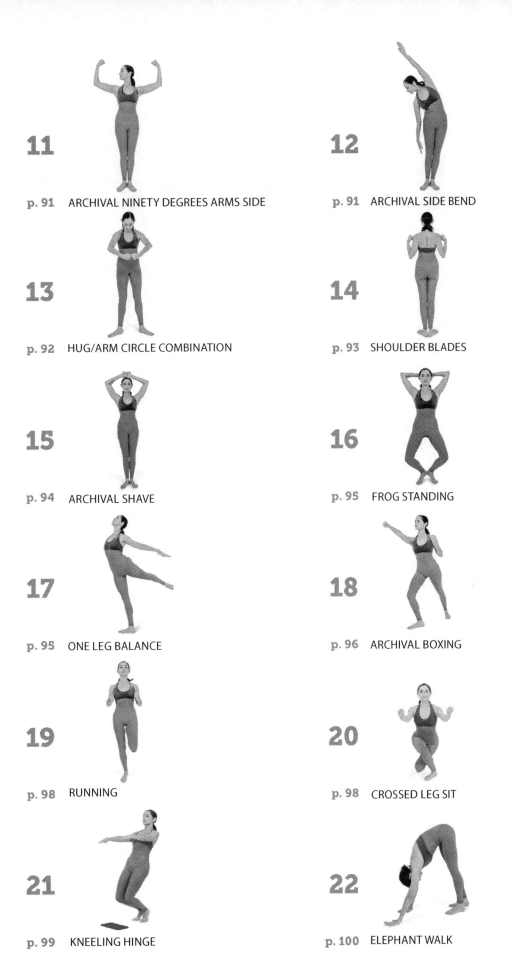

11   p. 91   ARCHIVAL NINETY DEGREES ARMS SIDE

12   p. 91   ARCHIVAL SIDE BEND

13   p. 92   HUG/ARM CIRCLE COMBINATION

14   p. 93   SHOULDER BLADES

15   p. 94   ARCHIVAL SHAVE

16   p. 95   FROG STANDING

17   p. 95   ONE LEG BALANCE

18   p. 96   ARCHIVAL BOXING

19   p. 98   RUNNING

20   p. 98   CROSSED LEG SIT

21   p. 99   KNEELING HINGE

22   p. 100   ELEPHANT WALK

JOE'S ARCHIVAL ROUTINE

INTRODUCTION

Joe's archival film footage inspired the exercise routine shown in this chapter *(Joseph H. Pilates: Demonstrating the Principles of his Method)*. Many of the archival exercises, like jumping jacks and jogging, did not originate with Joe Pilates, but this does not diminish their value. Joe took the time to document them with photos and films because he felt that they held an important place in his Method. In the film footage, Joe both taught and performed the exercises in a fairly consistent order. I have tried to represent that order here. With the exception of a few Matwork exercises near the beginning, most of the exercises are performed standing.

The majority of Joe's Archival Routine originated with the gymnastic-based strength training movement called Physical Culture, which was popular during the 19th century in Germany and other countries. My husband had a Physical Culture class as part of his general curriculum, as a child growing up in Russia. He recognized many of the exercises from his childhood when he watched the archival footage of Joe performing these routines. In addition to gymnastics, combat sports such as boxing, fencing, and wrestling also played a large role in the Physical Culture movement. Joe's background as a boxer, and his love of head wrestling, are also evident in the archival footage of his work.

You have the option of doing the full routine in the order described in this chapter, or you can focus on one or two standing exercises at the end of your Matwork routine.

JUMPING ROPE

Getting Started
You can learn this exercise with your hands on your hips, or with your arms in boxing position, hands made into fists, arms bent, and elbows pulled back slightly behind your waist. Starting with your feet together and powerhouse muscles activated, extend one leg forward with the foot above the floor and bend the supporting leg in preparation to hop onto the other leg. As you continue to hop from foot to foot, be sure that your back remains upright. Perform 1-2 sets of 8 hops.

Why It's Beneficial
The Jumping Rope exercise gets the blood pumping and warms up the body. It develops coordination and triggers the imagination.

Tips
Keep your weight on the balls of your feet and avoid locking your knees as you hop from foot to foot. Keep the movement fluid.

Eventually
Once you are coordinating the leg movement well, add arm movement that mimics the motion of turning a jump rope. Your elbows are tucked into your sides, your hands "hold" the jump rope handles with a loose grip, and your forearms and wrists move in very small circles going toward your body. Perform 1-2 sets of 8 hops. **Photos A-C**

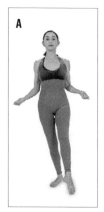 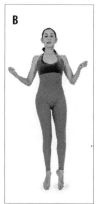 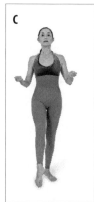

JUMPING JACKS

Getting Started

Stand with your feet together and powerhouse engaged. To perform the Jumping Jacks exercise with the arms in boxing position, make fists with your hands, bend your arms, and tuck your elbows into your sides. To open your chest, pull your elbows back slightly behind your waist. Jump your legs out slightly wider than your frame and jump your feet together again in a jumping jack pattern. Perform 10-20 sets. **Photos D-H**

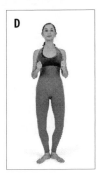 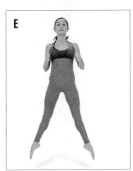 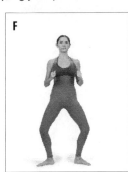 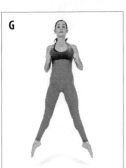 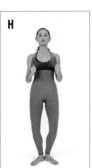

Why It's Beneficial

Jumping Jacks get the blood pumping and warm up the body. At the start of my daughter's lesson with a master Pilates teacher, she was given jumping jacks with the traditional up and down arm movement. I remember feeling surprised that the teacher would give her a "non-Pilates" exercise. After discovering the archival footage of Joe Pilates, I realized that she was giving an exercise from Joe's Archival Routine.

Tips

In the archival footage of Joe performing Jumping Jacks, he demonstrated three ways in which to position the arms: hands on the hips, arms in boxing position, or elbows tucked into the waist, wrists and forearms mimicking the motion of using a jump rope.

Distribute your weight evenly on both feet when landing from each jump. This is especially important when one foot is in front of the other.

Eventually

For an added challenge you can perform the entire Jumping Jacks sequence as taught by Joe:
  - Jump out slightly wider than hip bone width apart and jump the feet together again. Perform 5 sets. **Photos D-H**
  - Do small jumps with one leg in front and one leg behind for 6 repetitions (**Photos I-J**). Repeat with the other leg in front for about 6 repetitions (**Photo K**).
  - Alternate legs front and back while jumping about 8 times. **Photos I-K**
  - Jump with the feet together 8 times. **Photos L-M**

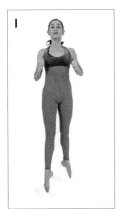 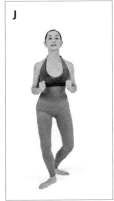 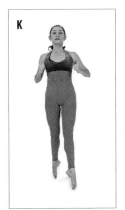 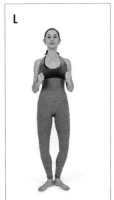 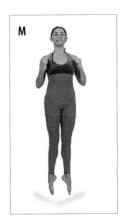

ROLL-UP

Joe Pilates describing the Roll-Up:

"Now start at the top of your head. Pretend you're a sack full of potatoes. Now let the potatoes roll out of you, one by one, until you're completely empty, an empty sack, empty of tensions, problems, troubles, and all the rest of it. You're just relaxing, letting go. The last potato is out and gone. Now start to fill up with new potatoes, new energy, health, happiness, prosperity, vitality. Are you finished? Are you full?"

Joe Pilates in Pageant

*See pages 74-75 in the Matwork with a Towel chapter for details on the Roll-Up. **Photos A-E**

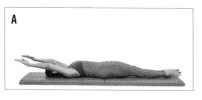
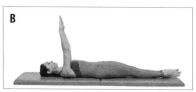
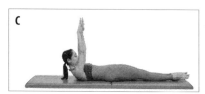
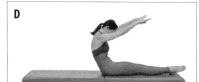
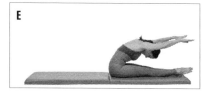

ROLL OVER

Getting Started

Lie on your back with your powerhouse engaged. You can draw your knees into your chest to help anchor your back. With your head still on the mat, extend your legs forward at working height, which is the lowest height at which you can keep your back anchored to the mat **(Photo F)**. Keeping your legs long and together, activate your powerhouse muscles and lift your legs up and over your head **(Photo G)**. Flex your feet with your legs together **(Photo H)**, then with your legs slightly wider than your frame **(Photo I)**. Keeping your legs apart, relax your feet **(Photo J)**, and roll down your spine with your thighs close to your chest **(Photo K)**. When you reach working height **(Photo L)**, draw your legs together **(Photo M)**. To reverse the sequence, open your legs as they go overhead and draw the legs together as you roll onto the mat. Perform 3 times starting with the legs together and 3 times starting with the legs apart.

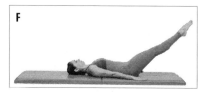
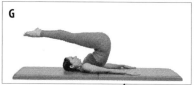
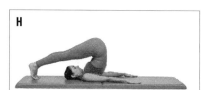
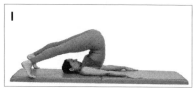
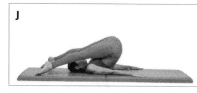
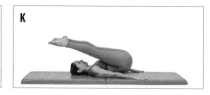

Why It's Beneficial

The Roll Over opens the low back, stretches the backs of the legs, and works the powerhouse muscles.

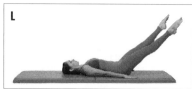
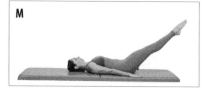

Tips

Initiate the lift of the hips from the powerhouse, not the legs. Keep the waistline lifted when the legs are overhead.

The Roll Over is an advanced exercise for students with healthy spines and strong powerhouse muscles. Omit this exercise if you have a delicate neck or back.

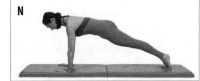

Eventually
To deepen the stretch in the backs of the legs at the end of each repetition, keep your feet flexed as you roll your spine onto the mat.

PUSH-UPS

After doing the Roll Over exercise, face the floor to perform Pilates Push-Ups with your elbows pointing toward your ribs as you bend your arms. See pages 50-51 in the Going Beyond Pre-Pilates for the Shoulders section of the Pre-Pilates chapter for details. **Photos N-O**

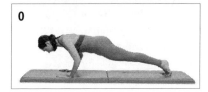

NOTE ABOUT THE LEG BICYCLE EXERCISE

Some of Joe's film footage documents the Leg Bicycle exercise performed in a shoulder stand at this point in the routine, and other parts of his film footage omits it. I've decided to omit it here because it is safer and more effective for most students to perform the Leg Bicycle exercise on the Small Barrel apparatus or the Spine Corrector. Romana also chose to omit the Leg Bicycle exercise from the Matwork routine for some students, choosing instead to perform it on the Small Barrel or Spine Corrector.

SAW STANDING

Getting Started
Stand with your feet apart and legs rotated outward from the hips. Extend your left arm toward the ceiling. Rotate from your waist, turning your torso to the right. Bend forward as you reach your left arm across your body, toward your right foot, and reach your other arm toward the ceiling. Roll up your spine as you take your left arm toward the ceiling again. Repeat on the other side. Perform 4 times. **Photos P-T**

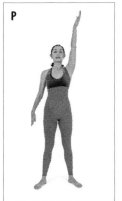
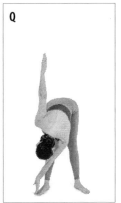
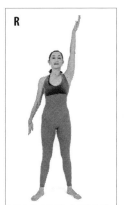
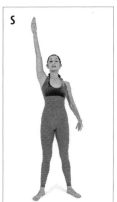
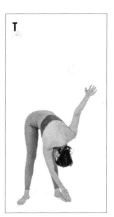

Why It's Beneficial
The Saw Standing works the sides of the body and stretches the backs of the legs.

Tips
To deepen the stretch, try to get your nose to your knee and your little finger to your little toe.

Eventually
Breathe in as you stand tall and breathe out as your hand reaches across your body, to the opposite foot. Breathing out on your twist will help you empty your lungs. Imagine that you are wringing out a wet towel as you rotate from your waist.

NOSE TO KNEE LUNGE

Getting Started

Stand with your feet apart and your legs rotated outward from the hips. Keep your arms long by your sides. Rotate from your waist, turning your torso to the right. Bend forward over your right leg. Your right leg bends as you bring your nose toward your knee. Roll up your spine to face forward. Repeat on the other side. Perform 4 times. **Photos A-D**

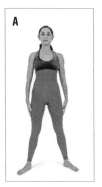 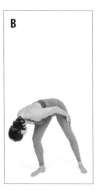 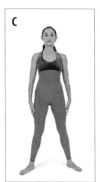 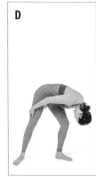

Why It's Beneficial

The Nose to Knee Lunge strengthens the legs and opens the low back.

Tips

Pay attention to the alignment of your knee as you bend your leg. Be sure to keep the middle of your knee in line with the middle of your foot.

Maintain a little daylight between your waist and your thigh as you bend your torso over each leg.

Eventually

Do the Nose to Knee Lunge to each side with your arms long by your sides **(Photos E-G)**. Next, extend your arms toward the ceiling as you lift your sternum **(Photo H)**. Soften your knees as you bend forward from your waist, swinging your arms between your legs **(Photo I)**. Roll up your spine with your arms long by your sides **(Photo J)**. Perform 2 sets.

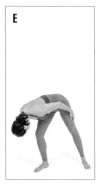 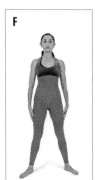 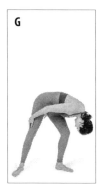 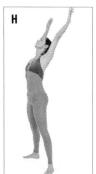 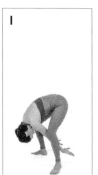 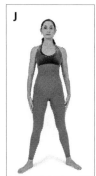

ARM SWINGING BACKBEND

Getting Started

Stand with your feet apart and powerhouse engaged. Extend your arms toward the ceiling and lift your sternum as you go into an upper backbend **(Photo K)**. Soften your knees and bend forward as you swing your arms between your legs **(Photo L)**. Perform 2 full sets.

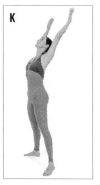 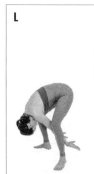

Why It's Beneficial

The Arm Swinging Backbend is a version of the Backbend exercise on the Ladder Barrel. It opens the chest and low back and limbers the spine.

Tips

To deepen the stretch, do three gentle pulses in the upper backbend with your arms overhead and in the forward bend with your arms between your legs.

Eventually

Once you are comfortable with the introductory variation of the Arm Swinging Backbend, add a deeper back extension with support from your hands. Lift your arms and sternum toward the ceiling **(Photo M)**. Then put your hands on your low back with your fingertips pointing to the floor as you go into a deeper backbend **(Photo N)**. Very flexible students can walk their hands

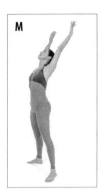 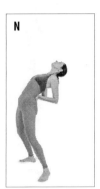 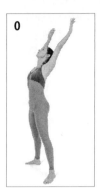 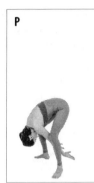

down the backs of their legs on the backbend. Roll up to standing and take your arms toward the ceiling **(Photo O)**. Soften your legs and swing your arms between your legs as you bend forward **(Photo P)**. Perform 2 sets.

HUGGING THE SUN

Getting Started

Stand with your arms down by your sides, feet close together, ideally in Pilates stance. Bend forward from your waist and reach for your toes **(Photo Q)**. Then extend your arms forward as you lift your torso parallel to the floor **(Photo R)**. Stand upright as your arms frame your face **(Photo S)**. As your arms open to the side, lift your chest toward the ceiling and go into an upper backbend **(Photo T)**. Lower your arms to complete the movement. Perform 3 times.

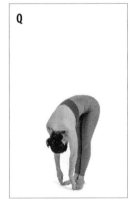 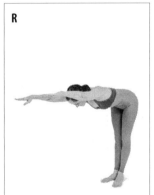 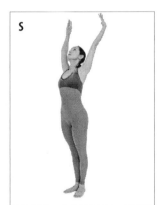 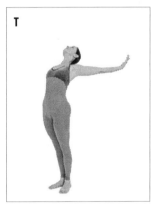

Why It's Beneficial

I fell in love with this archival exercise when I saw the footage of Joe performing and teaching it outdoors. It clearly has its roots in the Physical Culture movement that was popular when Joe was developing his method. My husband remembered doing an exercise called "Hugging the Sun" that looked just like this in Physical Culture classes when he was growing up in Russia. It is a very good stretch for the whole body, especially good for opening the low back and chest, and stretching the backs of the legs.

Tips

Imagine that you are diving into water as you reach for your toes. Remember to engage your powerhouse when you reach forward in the flat back position with your arms and torso parallel to the floor. As your arms open and your sternum lifts toward the ceiling, imagine that you are embracing the sun.

Eventually

This exercise can also be performed in reverse. Start each set with your arms forward at chest height, palms facing up **(Photo A)**. Lower your arms to your sides and reach back as your chest lifts toward the ceiling **(Photo B)**. From the upper backbend lift your arms above your head **(Photo C)** and bend forward, reaching toward your toes **(Photo D)**. Roll up to standing, arms long by your sides. Perform 3 times.

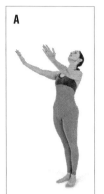 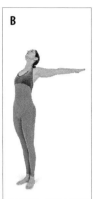 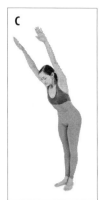 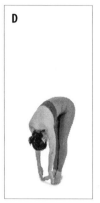

ORBITING THE SUN

Getting Started

This exercise is a variation of the Hugging the Sun exercise. It uses a spiral motion in the torso. You can practice this spiral motion before combining it with the Hugging the Sun sequence. Put your hands on your hips and bend your torso to one side, then spiral back and around to the other side and center. Repeat in the other direction. Learning this motion with your hands on your hips will help you focus on moving from your waist instead of moving from your arms.

Eventually

Once comfortable with the spiral motion from the waist as an individual exercise, you can incorporate it into the Hugging the Sun sequence. Stand with your arms down by your sides, feet close together, ideally in Pilates stance. Reach for your toes and extend your arms forward as you lift your torso parallel to the floor. From this flat back shape, sweep your arms and torso to one side, spiral back and around to the other side, and reach for your toes again. Perform 4 times with the spiral movement alternating direction each time. **Photos E-J**

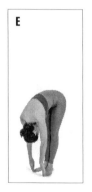 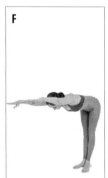 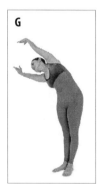 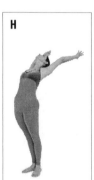 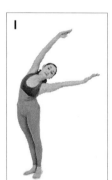 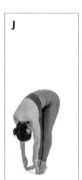

Tips

As you create the spiral motion with your upper body, imagine that your head is planet Earth orbiting the sun.

Why It's Beneficial

The Orbiting the Sun exercise stretches the backs of the legs, opens the low back and chest, and limbers the sides of the body.

ARCHIVAL NINETY DEGREES ARMS SIDE

Getting Started

Stand in Pilates stance and extend your arms to the side with your palms facing the ceiling. Without letting your elbows drop, form two fists and bend your arms. Each arm will form a right angle. Extend your arms to the side and up into a V-shape overhead with your palms facing down. Lower your arms to your legs, drop your gaze, and round your shoulders forward slightly to create a counter stretch. Perform 4 times.

Why It's Beneficial

The Archival Ninety Degrees Arms Side strengthens the upper arms, shoulders, and upper back.

Tips

To get the most from the exercise, create resistance as you move your arms through space, as though you are moving underwater.

Eventually

Add a neck stretch to complete the movement. Stand in Pilates stance with your arms to the side, palms facing the ceiling **(Photo K)**. Make fists as you form ninety-degree angles with your arms **(Photo L)**. Turn your head once over each shoulder **(Photos M-N)**. Extend your arms to the side and up into a V-shape overhead with your palms facing down **(Photo 0)**. Lower your arms to your legs, drop your gaze, and round your shoulders forward slightly to create a counter stretch **(Photo P)**. Perform 4 times.

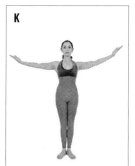 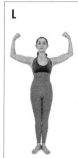 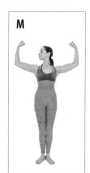 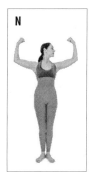 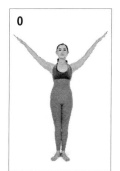 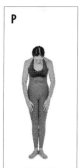

ARCHIVAL SIDE BEND

Getting Started

Stand with your feet together and extend your arms to the side **(Photo Q)**. Raise one arm toward your ear as your other arm stretches down by your leg **(Photo R)**. Go into a side bend, reaching away from the raised arm. Turn your head toward your bottom hand as you slide the palm of your hand down your leg **(Photo S)**. To come out of the side bend, center your torso, with your arms in a "V" shape overhead **(Photo T)**. To finish, lower your arms to your legs, drop your gaze, and round your shoulders forward slightly to create a counter stretch **(Photo U)**. Repeat on the other side. Perform 4 times.

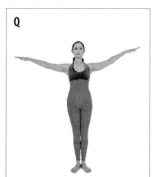 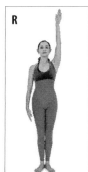 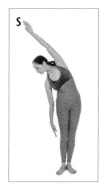 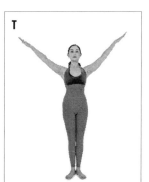 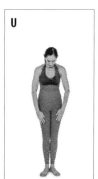

Why It's Beneficial
The Archival Side Bend stretches and strengthens the sides of the torso.

Tips
Keep your weight even on both feet as you bend your torso to each side.

Eventually
For an added challenge, you can do the Side Bend exercise from the Standing Weights series. Stand in Pilates stance with one to three pound weights in each

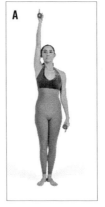
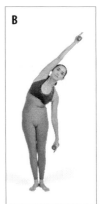
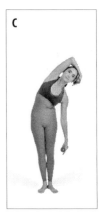

hand. Raise one arm toward your ear, leaving the other arm down by your side **(Photo A)**. Go into a side bend, reaching away from the raised arm **(Photo B)**. Keep your gaze straight ahead and fold your top arm around your head to deepen your stretch **(Photo C)**. While still in the side bend, stretch the top arm and center your torso. Repeat on the other side. Perform 4 times.

HUG/ARM CIRCLE COMBINATION

Getting Started
Stand with your feet apart and your legs rotated outward from the hips. Extend your arms to the side with your palms facing forward. Form fists as you draw your arms toward your midline, bend your arms into the closed hug shape, and round your shoulders forward slightly. Perform 4 times.

Eventually
Add an arm circle after each hug to complete the movement. Extend your arms to the side with your palms facing forward **(Photo D)**. After forming the closed hug shape **(Photo E)**, lift your arms and your sternum toward the ceiling **(Photo F)**. Turn your palms to the floor as they open to the side **(Photo G)**. Lower your arms to your legs, drop your gaze, and round your shoulders forward slightly to create a counter stretch **(Photo H)**. Perform 4 times.

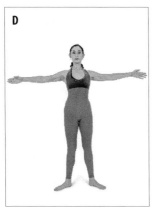
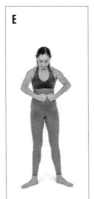
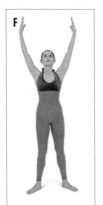
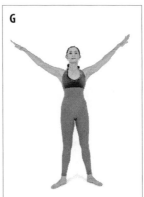
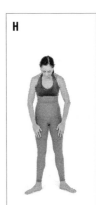

Why It's Beneficial
The Hug/Arm Circle Combination strengthens the arms and opens the chest.

Tips
As your arms extend to the side and your palms press down toward your legs, imagine that you are growing taller. Remember to create resistance as you move your arms through space.

SHOULDER BLADES

Getting Started

Stand in Pilates stance with your arms to the side, palms facing the ceiling **(Photo I)**. Without letting your elbows drop, form two fists and bend your arms all the way to each shoulder **(Photo J)**. Keeping your arms bent, slide your shoulder blades down your back as you pull your elbows down by your sides **(Photo K)**. Extend your arms in a V-shape overhead with your palms facing down **(Photo L)**. Lower your arms to your legs, drop your gaze, and round your shoulders forward slightly to create a counter stretch **(Photo M)**. Perform 4 times.

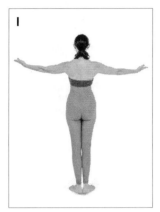 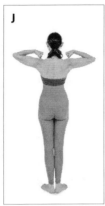 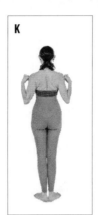 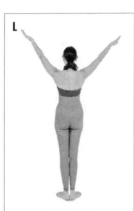 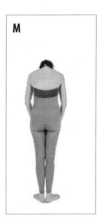

Why It's Beneficial

The Shoulder Blades exercise strengthens the back muscles and opens the chest.

Tips

To connect the arm movement to your back muscles, imagine that your shoulder blades are slippery bars of soap sliding down your back as you pull your arms down.

Eventually

To deepen the work in the upper back and increase the stretch in the chest, Joe taught the arm movement from the Double Leg Kick Matwork exercise in a standing posture. Stand in Pilates stance with your arms to the side, palms facing the floor **(Photo N)**. Bend your elbows and draw your hands behind you. Clasp one hand in the other near your upper back **(Photo O)**. Keeping your hands clasped, stretch your arms toward the floor as you lift your sternum toward the ceiling **(Photo P)**. Extend your arms in a V-shape overhead with your palms facing down **(Photo Q)**. Lower your arms to your legs, drop your gaze, and round your shoulders forward slightly to create a counter stretch **(Photo R)**. Perform 4 times.

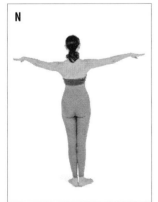 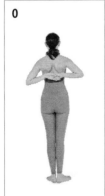 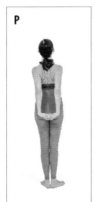 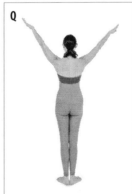 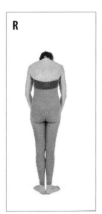

ARCHIVAL SHAVE

Getting Started

Standing in Pilates stance, extend your arms to the side with your palms facing the ceiling **(Photo A)**. Bring your hands above your head and clasp one hand in the other **(Photo B)**. Pull your clasped hands down onto the crown of your head as your elbows press open **(Photo C)**. Keeping your hands clasped, stretch your arms toward the ceiling **(Photo D)**. Pull your hands down onto the crown of your head as your elbows press open one more time **(Photo E)**. Stretch your arms up as the arms separate into a V-shape overhead with the palms facing each other **(Photo F)**. Lower your arms to your legs, drop your gaze, and round your shoulders forward slightly to create a counter stretch **(Photo G)**. Perform 4 times.

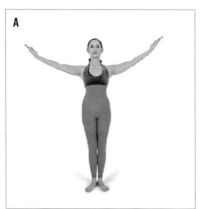
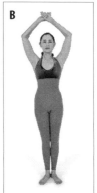
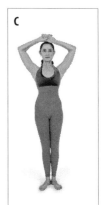

Why It's Beneficial

The Archival Shave exercise opens the chest and shoulders, and strengthens the arms and upper back.

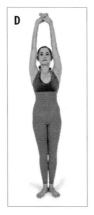
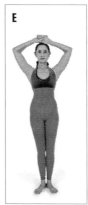
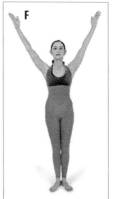
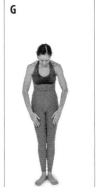

Tips

To get the best stretch in your chest, don't move your head as you move your arms. Keep your gaze straight ahead and press your elbows open as your pull your hands down onto the crown of your head.

Remember to create resistance as you move your arms through space.

Eventually

The Standing Weights version of the Shave intensifies the stretch in the chest and shoulders. Stand in Pilates stance with one to three pound weights in each hand. Your arms are in front of your legs with the ends of the weights together **(Photo H)**. Keeping the weights together, bend your elbows to the side and draw them up your body's midline **(Photo I)**. Keeping the elbows open, bring the weights over and behind your head, toward the base of your skull **(Photo J)**. Keeping the weights together, stretch your arms toward the ceiling on a slight diagonal forward **(Photo K)**. Bend your arms behind your head and stretch your arms up on a forward diagonal 2 to 4 more times. Lower your arms in the front of your legs to finish.

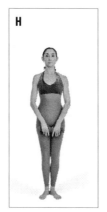
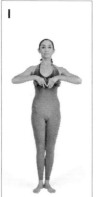
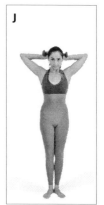
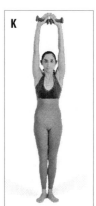

FROG STANDING

Getting Started

Stand in Pilates stance and open your arms to the side, palms facing the ceiling **(Photo L)**. Stack your hands behind your head **(Photo M)**. With your powerhouse lifted, imagine that your back is sliding down a pole as you bend your legs **(Photo N)**. At a certain point, your heels lift off the floor reluctantly **(Photo O)**. Go into the deepest knee bend appropriate for your body **(Photo P)**. When you are ready to straighten your legs, push your heels onto the floor as soon as you can, without sticking your seat out. After performing 2 Knee Bends, open your arms out in a V-shape overhead **(Photo Q)**. Lower your arms by your sides to finish.

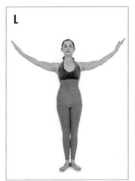 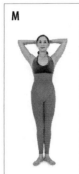 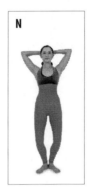 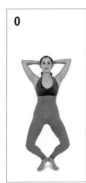 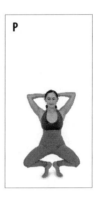 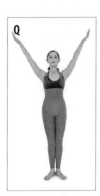

Why It's Beneficial

The Frog Standing strengthens the legs and bottom, and improves posture and balance.

Tips

Press the back of your head into your hands, as your hands resist the pressure. Creating opposing lines of energy between the hands and the back of the head will help you maintain length in the back of your neck and keep your chest lifted, and will prevent you from sticking your seat out as you bend and straighten your knees.

This exercise is not appropriate for students with knee issues.

Eventually

For an added challenge, start on the half toe and perform three pauses as you bend your knees, and three pauses as you stretch your legs. After performing 2 Knee Bends, open your arms out in a V-shape overhead, and lower your arms to your sides as you lower your heels to the floor.

ONE LEG BALANCE

Getting Started

Stand with your feet together in parallel, or in Pilates stance. As you open your arms to the side, extend one leg forward. Try to hold your balance on one leg for at least three counts. Repeat on the other side. Perform 4 times. **Photo R**

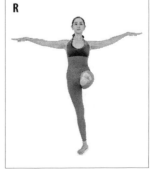

Why It's Beneficial

The One Leg Balance improves balance control, stretches the working leg, and strengthens the supporting leg. It challenges you to maintain evenness in your hips and shoulders as your body weight shifts from two feet to one.

Tips

Remember to pull up through your standing hip and thigh as your working leg extends in the air.

Eventually

When you are ready, raise your leg to the side as your arms open. To avoid looking like a dog at a fire hydrant as your leg lifts, try to rotate your inner thigh toward the ceiling. Repeat on the other side. Perform 4 times. **Photo S**

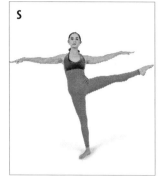 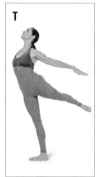

For an added challenge, try to lift your leg straight out to the back as you extend your arms to the side. While in this shape, which is called an *arabesque* in ballet, mimic the arm movement from the "T" on the Reformer, opening your arms wider and lifting your sternum higher. To deepen the stretch in the chest, pulse your arms back toward your back leg as you hold them out to the side. Imagine that you are cracking a walnut between your shoulder blades as your arms pulse back. Repeat on the other side. Perform 2 sets. **Photo T**

ARCHIVAL BOXING
Getting Started

Joe Pilates was an avid boxer, as this next sequence of exercises clearly demonstrates. As this is not a book written specifically for boxers, these exercises are described in very simple terms. Details, such as raising the shoulder of the boxing arm as a means of protecting the chin, and pivoting the back foot on certain punches as a means of gaining more power have been left out. If you are familiar with boxing technique, feel free to incorporate more details.

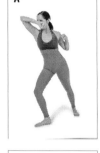

Starting Position: Start in a forward lunge with the right leg in front and the left leg in back. Shift your weight forward and bend your front leg. Guard your face with your right arm crossed in front of your face. Tuck your left elbow down by your side. **Photo A**

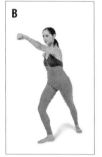 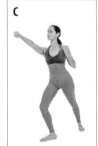

Variation One: This variation is inspired by two types of *straight punches,* the *cross punch* and the *jab.* After going into starting position with your right leg in front, punch first with your left arm, then with your right arm. Perform 2-4 times. Repeat on the other side with the left leg in front. **Photos B-C**

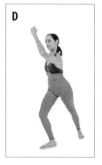 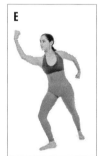

Variation Two: This variation is inspired by two types of *round punches,* the *back uppercut* and the *lead uppercut.* After going into starting position with your right leg in front, stretch your left arm behind you in preparation to punch your left arm forward in an upward motion. Your left arm is bent with the elbow down and the back of your hand is facing away from you. Repeat with your right arm. You can soften your knees as you perform the punches. Perform 2-4 times. Repeat on the other side with the left leg in front. **Photos D-E**

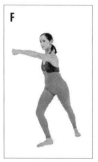 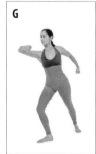

Variation Three: This variation is inspired by two types of *round punches,* the *back hook* and the *lead hook.* After going into starting position with your right leg in front, stretch your left arm behind you in preparation to punch your left arm around to the front. Your left arm is bent with the elbow lifted to the side, palm facing toward you. Repeat with your right arm. Perform 2-4 times. Repeat on the other side with the left leg in front. **Photos F-G**

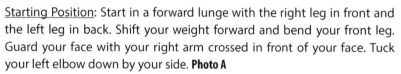

<u>Variation Four:</u> This variation is inspired by the *overhand punch,* a semi-circular punch thrown with the rear hand. After going into starting position with your right leg in front, stretch your left arm behind you in preparation to punch your left arm around to the front with the back of your hand turned toward the midline, palm facing out. Repeat with your right arm. Perform 2-4 times. Repeat on the other side with the left leg in front. **Photos H-I**

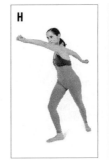 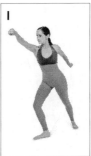

Why It's Beneficial
The Archival Boxing exercise strengthens the arms. *When done with special attention to boxing technique,* it can be good for self-defense

Tips
To make the punches more realistic, don't keep your legs and torso static as you punch. Let the body move with the arm as it punches, softening the knees, pivoting the back foot, and twisting from the hips.

Eventually
After learning the four boxing variations separately, perform them in succession. Perform 2-4 of each variation. **Photos J-U**

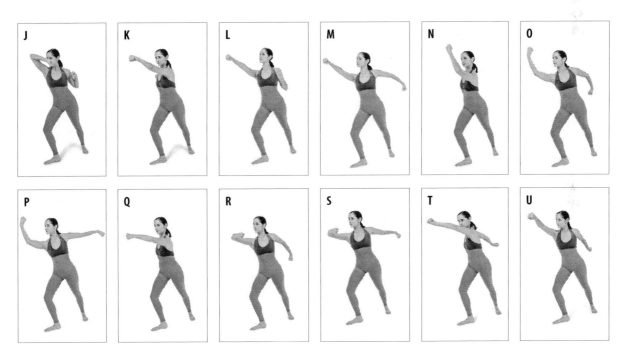

RUNNING

Getting Started

Stand with your feet close together. Form fists, bend your arms, and tuck your elbows into your sides. To open your chest, pull your elbows slightly behind your waist. Jog in place while kicking your heels toward your seat **(Photo A)**. Next, stack your forearms, lift your elbows, and jog in place with one knee lifting toward your chest with each weight shift **(Photo B)**. Perform 8 heel kicks to the seat and 8 knee lifts to the front. Repeat up to 2 more sets.

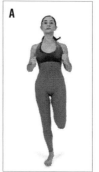 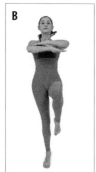

Why It's Beneficial

The Running exercise gets the heart rate up, increases the blood circulation, improves endurance, and is fun.

Tips

The Running exercise should be done near the end of the lesson, when you are sufficiently warmed up and the backs of your legs are limber.

Eventually

If space allows, run the perimeter of the room while trying to kick your heels toward your seat. Next, cross your arms "genie" style and run another set of laps as you lift your knees toward your chest. The number of laps will vary, depending on your ability level and the amount of space you have to work in.

CROSSED LEG SIT

"So you want to learn. Lie down on the mat.
Don't flop down, go down smoothly, like this, cross the arms, cross the legs."
Joe Pilates in *Sports Illustrated*

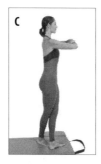 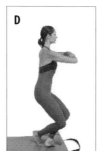 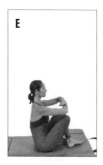

Getting Started

Stand in Pilates stance with your arms stretched forward, palms facing up. Keeping the weight primarily on the front foot, cross one leg behind you, and bend your legs as you sink to the floor. Keeping your arms away from the floor, stand up. Repeat with the other leg crossing behind. Perform 2-4 times. **Photos F-I**

Why It's Beneficial

The Crossed Leg Sit strengthens the legs and develops the poise and control necessary to lower oneself to the floor.

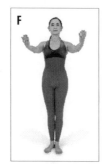 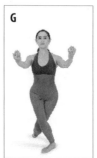 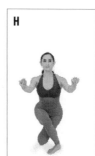 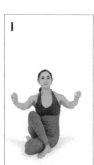

This exercise is not appropriate for students with delicate knees.

Eventually
The Crossed Leg Sit can be performed with the weight more evenly distributed between both legs. This is the variation that is used at the start of a Matwork routine performed on the floor. Stand in Pilates stance with your arms long by your sides or with your forearms crossed and elbows lifted. Cross one foot in front of the other and sink to the floor to sit, without putting your hands on the floor. Stand up without letting your hands touch the floor. Repeat with the other leg crossing in front. Perform 2-4 times. **Photos C-E or Photos J-N**

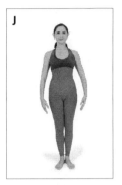 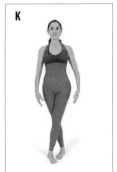 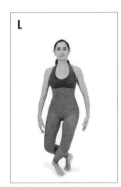 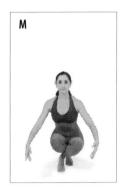 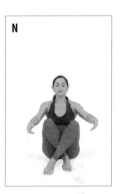

KNEELING HINGE

Getting Started
Place a pad on the floor in front of you. Stand behind the pad with your feet close together. Try to keep your pelvis forward and your chest lifted as you lower your knees to the floor while raising your arms to shoulder level in front of you. With your toes curled under, stand up as you lift your arms toward the ceiling. Perform 2 times. **Photos O-T**

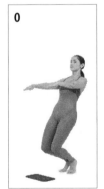 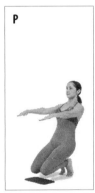 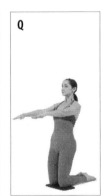 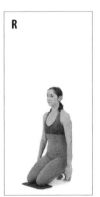 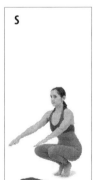 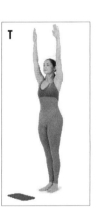

Why It's Beneficial
The Kneeling Hinge strengthens the legs and develops the poise and control necessary to lower oneself to the floor.

Tips
This exercise is not appropriate for students with delicate knees or toe joints.

Eventually
Once you have mastered the Kneeling Hinge, add a variation that opens the chest and works the lungs. After kneeling on the floor, uncurl your toes, put your hands on the floor in front of you, and slide your hands forward as you lengthen your spine. Keep your elbows and your bellybutton lifted above the mat as you lift your sternum toward the ceiling and breathe out. Lower your head and slide your hands back toward your knees. Curl your toes under and stand up as you lift your arms. Perform 2 times. **Photos A-J**

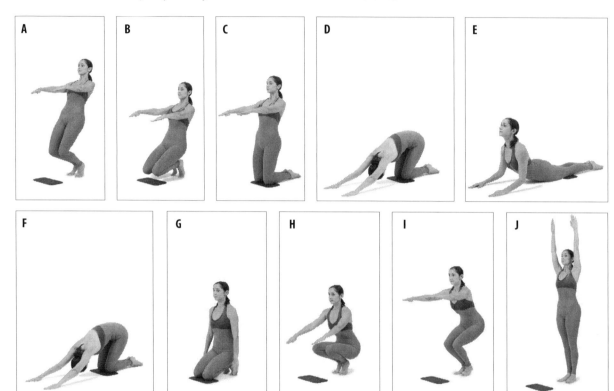

ELEPHANT WALK

Getting Started
Stand with your feet parallel and hip width apart. Bend forward and try to place your fingertips, and if possible, your palms, on the floor in front of your feet. Your head is hanging, waistline lifted, and limbs as long as possible. Step forward with your right arm and leg, followed by your left arm and leg, and continue walking in this pattern with minimal bending in your knees and elbows. Take 6-8 steps forward, bring your feet together and roll through your spine to stand tall. **Photo K**

Why It's Beneficial
The Elephant Walk opens the low back, stretches the backs of the legs, strengthens the stomach, and improves coordination.

Tips
Pull your bellybutton and ribs up toward the ceiling as you take each step. Engaging your powerhouse muscles makes it easier to walk on all fours.

Eventually
As your powerhouse strength, flexibility, and coordination improve, try the Elephant Walk in reverse.

WORKS CITED

Brown, Beth. "How to Stay Fit Lying Down." *Pageant,* Nov. 1963, pp. 128-133.

Joseph H. Pilates: Demonstrating the Principles of his Method with Clara, Students and Friends. Archival film footage compiled and edited by Mary Bowen from Joe Pilates' private film collection, 1932-1945.

Wernick, Robert. "To Keep in Shape: Act Like an Animal." *Sports Illustrated,* Eastern Edition, 12 Feb. 1962, pp. E5-E8.

Romana's Standing Exercises

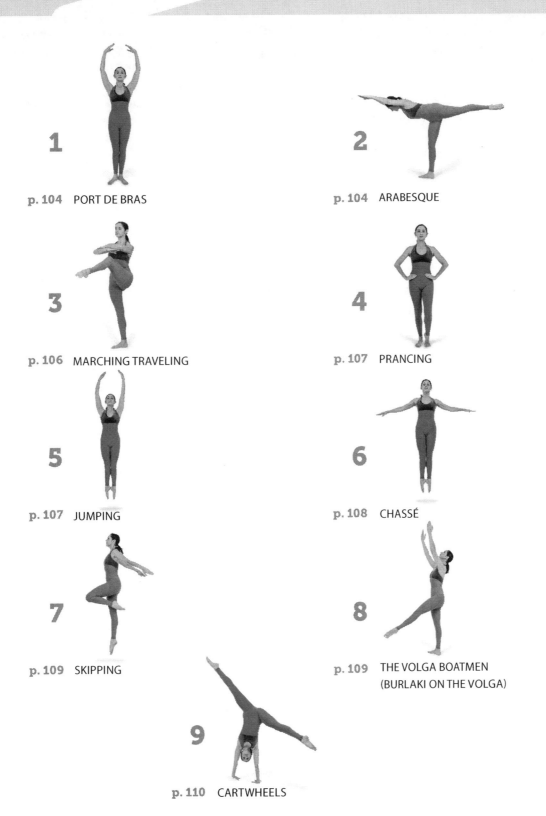

1

p. 104   PORT DE BRAS

2

p. 104   ARABESQUE

3

p. 106   MARCHING TRAVELING

4

p. 107   PRANCING

5

p. 107   JUMPING

6

p. 108   CHASSÉ

7

p. 109   SKIPPING

8

p. 109   THE VOLGA BOATMEN
          (BURLAKI ON THE VOLGA)

9

p. 110   CARTWHEELS

ROMANA'S STANDING EXERCISES

INTRODUCTION

In addition to teaching Pilates, Joe Pilates' protégé, Romana Kryzanowska taught ballet classes to young children. She was known for bringing a child-like playfulness into the Pilates studio. It was quite normal to see a group of Romana's adult students skipping across her studio as if they were children in a creative movement class. I loved it when Romana used a play-based approach to movement, because it lightened the mood and left my body feeling invigorated. While skipping and cartwheels did not originate with Romana or Joe, Romana saw the value of using them with many of her Pilates students. You can practice an entire cluster of these exercises, or you can concentrate on just one or two. Romana's Standing Exercises are a valuable addition to your personal practice because they offer a freedom of movement that will take your Pilates skills to the next level. Any of these exercises would be a fun addition at the end of your workout.

PORT DE BRAS

Getting Started

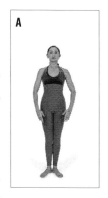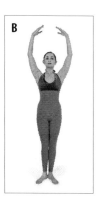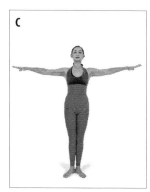

Port de Bras is a French ballet term that means "carriage of the arms." To perform the Port de Bras exercise, stand with your feet close together, in the stance appropriate for your body, arms in front of your thighs **(Photo A)**. Activate your powerhouse muscles and begin to inhale as you lift your arms in front of you in the closed hug position. As you continue to inhale, your arms lift higher, until they frame your face **(Photo B)**. As you breathe out, your arms open to the side, palms facing the floor, arms staying within your field of vision **(Photo C)**. Perform 3 arm circles.

Why It's Beneficial

Romana used to give the Port de Bras exercise at the end of a lesson. It has a calming, yet energizing effect. It centers the body, works the breath, lifts the powerhouse, and serves as a nice cool down.

Tips

Creating opposing lines of energy is particularly useful in this exercise. As your arms press down on the exhalation, remember to pull up through your body. Imagine that your head is a cork lifting out of a wine bottle and your arms are the levers of a corkscrew pressing toward the floor.

Eventually

For an added challenge, rise onto the half toe as you breathe in, lifting your arms forward and up. On the exhalation, lower your heels to the floor with control as you lower your arms out to the side. Perform 3 arm circles.

ARABESQUE

Getting Started

Arabesque is a ballet term that describes a one-legged posture in which a dancer extends one leg behind him and raises it off the floor. To perform the Arabesque exercise, stand with your powerhouse lifted and your feet close to each other, in the stance appropriate for you body **(Photo D)**. Raise your arms toward the ceiling until they frame your face, and extend one leg behind you in the arabesque pose **(Photos E-F)**. As your leg continues

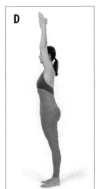 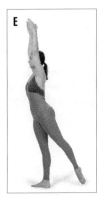 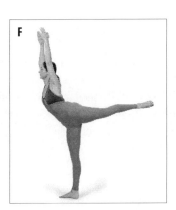 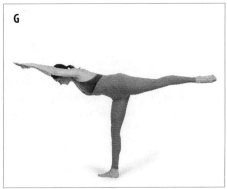

to lift behind you, your torso begins to tip forward with your arms reaching forward. Your body forms the letter "T" with your arms and raised leg parallel to the floor (Photo G). Hold the "T" shape for three to five seconds before returning to the starting position with both feet on the floor. Perform 2 times on each leg.

Why It's Beneficial

The Arabesque exercise is inspired by the Pilates Push-Ups performed on one leg in the Matwork. It develops powerhouse stability, improves balance, and strengthens the supporting hip.

Tips

It is tempting to put all the focus on the standing leg while trying to balance, but if there is no energy in the raised leg, achieving a steady balance can feel almost impossible. To gain more stability as you balance on one leg, remember to reach out through the toes of your raised leg.

Eventually

As you gain balance control, you can increase the range of movement in the raised leg. After going into the "T" shape, continue to lift your back leg toward the ceiling as your torso reluctantly tips forward. When your leg has reached your maximum height, gently place your hands on the floor. Your head is tucked in as you lift your waist toward the ceiling. The shape is similar to the Arabesque exercise on the Reformer. **Photo H**

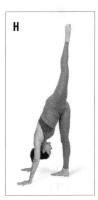

For an additional challenge, with your hands still on the floor, lift your bellybutton and your raised leg toward the ceiling as your supporting foot rises up onto the half toe (Photo I). Lower your supporting heel to the floor and begin to lift your hands off the floor (Photo J). Extend your arms forward and lift your torso, creating the "T" shape again (Photo K). With your back leg still raised, try to lift your torso upright before placing your back foot on the floor (Photo L). Finish the exercise standing on both feet with your arms reaching toward the ceiling (Photo M). Perform 1 time on each leg.

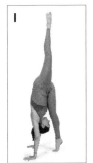 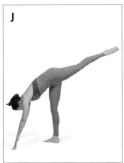 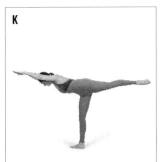 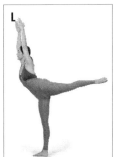 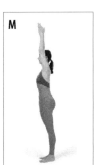

MARCHING TRAVELING

Getting Started

Unlike the Pre-Pilates variation of the Marching exercise, which is performed standing in place, the Marching Traveling exercise moves across the room. Standing with your forearms crossed and elbows lifted, or with arms extended to the side, brush the ball of your foot forward on the floor before lifting your bent knee. This approach to lifting the leg is similar to a *grand battement* movement in ballet. Step forward each time you bring the kicking leg down to the floor. **Photos N-S**

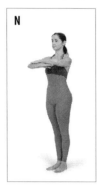 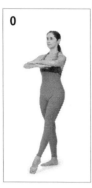 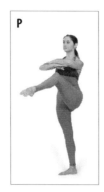 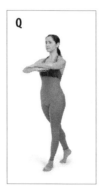 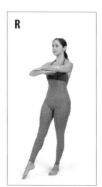 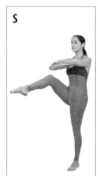

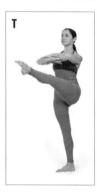

For an extra stretch, keep your leg straight as you brush it forward and lift it off the floor **(Photo T)**.

Perform about 20 knee lifts or straight kicks traveling forward.

Why It's Beneficial

The Marching Traveling exercise develops balance control, strengthens the supporting hip, and stretches the muscles in the working leg and hip.

Tips

Make sure that your heel stays along the midline as you travel forward.

Eventually

The Marching Traveling can also be done with the leg lifting to the side. To perform Marching Traveling with side leg lifts, stand in Pilates stance facing the front of the room, arms extended to the side **(Photo U)**. Brush your foot across the floor to the side and lift your bent knee toward your arm **(Photo V)**. Step out onto the kicking foot and pivot on that foot as you turn toward the back of the room. Repeat the knee lift with your other foot brushing across the floor to the side, lifting your bent knee toward your arm. To keep the movement traveling in one direction, always turn toward the foot that comes back to the floor from the side knee lift.

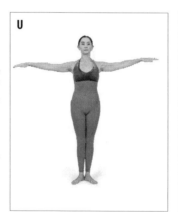 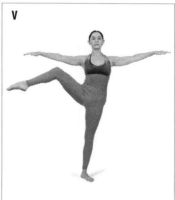

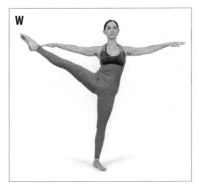
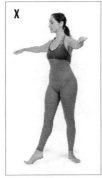
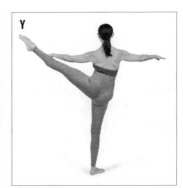
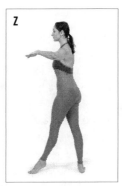

For an extra stretch, keep your leg straight as you brush it out to the side and lift it off the floor. **Photos W-Z**

Perform about 20 knee lifts or straight kicks traveling across the room to the right. Repeat the sideways movement to the left.

PRANCING

Getting Started

Stand with your feet and legs parallel and slightly apart and your hands on your hips. With your powerhouse lifted, rise onto the half toe **(Photo AA)**. As you lower one heel to the floor, keeping your leg straight, the other leg bends, keeping that foot on the half toe **(Photo BB)**. Alternate lifting the heels 20 times with the accent on the upbeat. The up is when both legs are straight with the heels lifted.

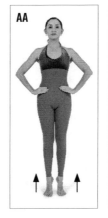
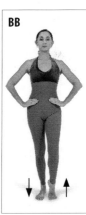

Why It's Beneficial

The Prancing exercise works the feet and calves and promotes correct body placement in the upright position, with weight forward on the balls of the feet and light on the heels.

Tips

You will have improved balance and control if you focus on using your powerhouse to lift your heels. Remember to lengthen your spine and pull your bellybutton up each time you move your ankles. Imagine that your bellybutton is a yo-yo and your spine is the string.

Eventually

For a deeper stretch in the calves and Achilles tendons, you can do the Prancing exercise with the balls of your feet on the edge of a thick book or the edge of a step. In the beginning, you may need to hold something stable for balance. But the goal is to do the Prancing exercise with the arms long by the sides of the body. The sooner you don't have anything to rely on for balance assistance, the sooner you learn to adjust your posture to maintain balance and control.

JUMPING

Getting Started

Learn to coordinate the movement in your arms and legs before adding the jumping motion. Stand in the stance appropriate for your body with your arms down by your sides. Lift through your powerhouse as you bend your knees over your toes with your heels on the floor. This is a *plié* position in ballet. When you stretch your legs, swing your arms forward. Then bend your legs again as your arms come down by your sides. The second time you stretch your legs, swing your arms behind you. Practice swinging the arms forward and backward in unison with straightening the legs, until you are comfortable with the rhythm of the movement.

Eventually

After you are used to swinging your arms every time you straighten your legs, you can start jumping. Begin with your feet close to each other in the stance that best suits your body. Go into the *plié* position with the middle of each knee in line with the middle of each foot. To maintain the lift in your powerhouse, imagine that you are getting taller as you bend your legs. When you push off for your jump, imagine that you are being sucked through a vacuum cleaner that is being held above your head. As you take off for the first jump, your arms begin to swing forward as you "zip" up your inner thighs **(Photos CC-DD)**. After landing, you rebound into the air with your arms swinging back **(Photos EE-FF)**. Alternate the direction of the arms on each jump. Perform up to 20 jumps.

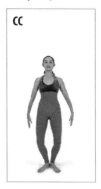 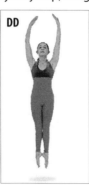 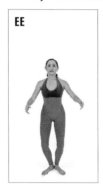 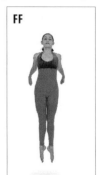

Why It's Beneficial

The Jumping exercise strengthens the legs and seat muscles. It is a good exercise for athletes who need to improve the elevation of their jumps. Jumping is also quite fun. Jumping improves the circulation of oxygen-rich blood to the brain, which tends to positively influence one's mood and creativity. It is a good choice for a final exercise in a workout. Romana often gave this exercise at the end of the Matwork routine.

Tips

Good elevation in jumps requires powerful gluteal muscles, and that power can only be achieved with the correct footing on the ground. Getting the heels down on the ground when landing from each jump will give you more power to push off for the next jump. There is a powerful connection between pushing off the floor with the whole foot and using the gluteal muscles to get elevation.

Keeping the back upright when landing from each jump can be challenging. Remember to engage your powerhouse muscles to help stabilize your torso.

To determine if your jumps are staying in one spot, place a thin pad on the floor and try to land from each of your jumps on the pad.

CHASSÉ

Getting Started

Stand with your arms held out to the side. Extend your right leg to the side and step onto it as you bend your legs slightly and jump with both legs together in the air. After landing on your left leg, repeat consecutive jumps to the right. When done correctly, it appears as though the left leg is chasing the right leg. Repeat on the other side. **Photos GG-II**

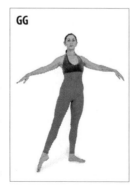 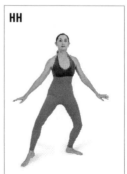 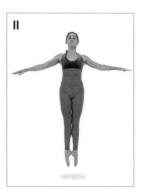

Why It's Beneficial

A *chassé* is a ballet movement that means "chase" in French. But this movement is not only performed in a ballet setting. Many baseball players, basketball players, and other athletes use it as part of their warm-up routine. The Chassé exercise gets the blood circulating and warms up the body. It also works the inner thighs as the legs come together in the air.

Tips

Many years ago, my husband and I won a free ballroom dance lesson. My husband did not want to tell our teacher that we were former professional ballet dancers, so we ended up having a very basic class. During the class, the teacher compared the leg movement in a *chassé* to the leg movement of a person trying to pass through a narrow movie aisle on his way to get popcorn. Although it was a silly image for us as former professional dancers, it is the perfect image for those learning the movement for the first time.

Eventually

Once the coordination of the legs is established, add arm movement. Start with your arms to the side as you take your first step. Your forearms cross each other in front of your body on the first jump, and on the next jump you open your arms out to the side. Continue to alternate swinging the arms to the crossed position and the stretched position. Perform in both directions.

SKIPPING

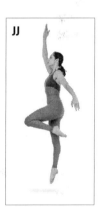

Getting Started

In the skipping movement, the arm opposite the bent leg reaches toward the ceiling on every skip. When you learn skipping with one arm up in the air with each skip, you probably won't have to focus on which arm should go up. Just as most people naturally use the arm opposite the leading foot when walking, most people naturally use the arm opposite the raised knee when skipping. **Photo JJ**

Why It's Beneficial

Romana was an expert at getting us to run, skip, and jump around the studio like children. Skipping develops coordination and endurance and is fun.

Tips

Put the emphasis on the height of the jump instead of on traveling forward.

Eventually

For variety, alternate lifting and lowering both arms as you skip. Lifting your arms toward the ceiling helps you focus on gaining elevation.
Photos KK-NN

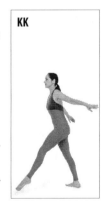 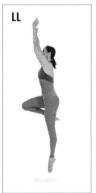 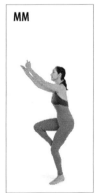 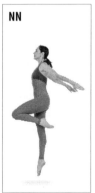

THE VOLGA BOATMEN (BURLAKI ON THE VOLGA)

Note

I owe a big thank you to my husband, who was born and raised in Russia, for sharing the details about the Russian music, art, and history that inspired Romana to create this exercise.

Getting Started

Learn the Volga Boatmen exercise with the arms stationary and held out to the side to help with balance. Stand in the stance that suits your body and brush one foot forward along the floor until your leg is a few inches above the floor in front of you. Try to hold your balance for four counts before stepping forward into a lunge with the front leg bent for another four counts. Make sure that your front foot lands with control as the toes, ball of the foot, and heel go to the floor. After holding this forward lunge for four counts, repeat the movement on the other side. Continue alternating sides while traveling across the room.

Eventually

Once you have a steady balance, add the upper body movement. As you extend your leg forward, extend your arms forward and lift them toward the ceiling. Hold your leg in the air with your sternum lifted for four counts **(Photo 00)**. As you step onto the front leg in a forward lunge, lower your head and place your hands on the floor **(Photo PP)**. Continue alternating sides while traveling across the room.

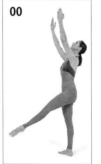 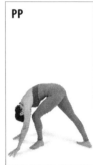

Why It's Beneficial

Romana took her inspiration for this exercise from the famous Russian painting entitled *Barge Haulers on the Volga* by Ilya Repin. This exercise is a reenactment of the painting that depicts a team of laborers, known as burlaki in Russian, towing a boat along the bank of the Volga River. When teaching this exercise, Romana had us imagine that we were doing the backbreaking work of the burlaki, who dragged barges upstream with a tow rope.

Romana created this exercise to give students the opportunity to move with freedom across the floor, while challenging their balance control. It helps people use their imagination and teaches them a little about Russian culture, too!

Tips

For me, the best part of this exercise was performing it as Romana hummed the famous Russian folk song that became associated with the painting. *The Song of the Volga Boatmen* helped us synchronize our steps, and taught those with little or no music experience how to count music. If you look up this song on the Internet, you can hum the tune as you perform the exercise.

Before it became associated with the painting, Russian peasants sang this song as they cleared land for crops and built homes. The music helped them coordinate their movements as they pulled ropes to uproot trees and hammered poles into the ground. The lyrics to this famous song, translate as: *"Yo, Heave Ho! Yo, Heave Ho!"* and *"Mighty stream so deep and wide. Volga, Volga you're our pride."* The lyrics illustrate both the appeals to pull harder, and the dignity of these proud laborers. In this exercise, Romana beautifully reflected the extremes illustrated in the song. Pride and respect for the Volga River is represented with raised arms and the chest lifted toward the sky. Exhaustion from engaging in heavy, repetitive work is represented with a forward lunge with the head down and hands on the ground.

CARTWHEELS

Tips

This exercise requires balance control and upper body strength. Before adding cartwheels to your workout, be sure you are comfortable with the Arabesque exercise on pages 104-105 of this chapter, and with the L-Shape on the Wall exercise described on page 51 in the Going Beyond Pre-Pilates for the Shoulders section of the Pre-Pilates chapter.

Getting Started

While some people do a side bend to go into a cartwheel, a true cartwheel should start with the body bending forward. To do a cartwheel on your dominant side, extend your arms toward the ceiling and raise your dominant leg forward **(Photo QQ)**. After extending your leg front, go into a forward lunge with your front leg bent and your back leg straight. Raise your back leg so that it is parallel to the floor and your arms and torso reach forward so that they are also parallel to the floor. From the "T" shape, lift your back leg higher so that you tip forward **(Photo RR)**. When your hands go to the floor they are turned at a right angle to your front foot. Kick your legs over your head one at a time, starting with your back leg **(Photo SS)**. The foot that kicked first lands first **(Photo TT)**. Finish the cartwheel in a lunge facing the opposite direction from which you began.

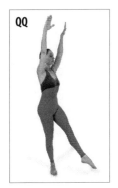
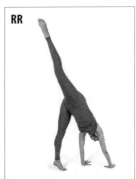
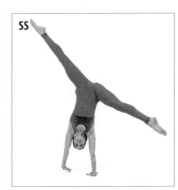
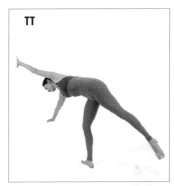

Why It's Beneficial

Cartwheels strengthen the arms, shoulders, and back muscles. They develop balance, coordination, and improve spatial awareness.

Eventually

When you are comfortable performing your cartwheel to each side, you can perform consecutive cartwheels across the room. Please note that you land from each cartwheel in a lunge facing the opposite direction to which you are traveling, and have to rotate your body toward your back foot to continue cartwheeling in the direction in which you began.

About the Author

A dual citizen of Brazil and the United States, Christina Maria Gadar has the distinction of having been trained and certified directly under Joseph Pilates' original protégé, Romana Kryzanowska. Christina was introduced to the Pilates Method at the age of fifteen while a student at the Boston Ballet.

During her ballet training she was coached privately for six years by acclaimed ballet dancer and Baryshnikov rival, Fernando Bujones. After receiving dance scholarships from the Massachusetts Arts Council and the School of the Boston Ballet, she went on to dance professionally with many ballet companies, including the Sarasota Ballet of Florida, where she met her husband.

Christina has specialized in private instruction of the original Pilates Method since 2000. She discovered her love for Pre-Pilates Exercises, Towel Exercises, and Standing Pilates Exercises while developing the syllabus for *Pilates for Children*, a book she wrote for teachers interested in teaching Pilates to children. She has discovered that writing about Pilates, in addition to teaching the Method, is a fulfilling way to expand her passion for Pilates.

Christina enjoys the balancing act of running her Pilates studio with the highest standards while writing and staying actively involved in the lives of her family, including her two children and many pets.

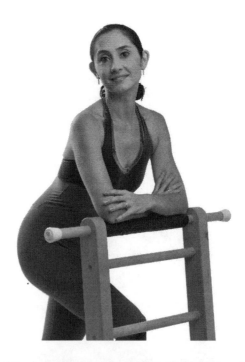

"We delight in the beauty of the butterfly, but rarely admit the changes it has gone through to achieve that beauty."

Maya Angelou
in *Rainbow in the Cloud: The Wisdom and Spirit of Maya Angelou,* 2014.

Made in the USA
Columbia, SC
10 June 2022

61579178R00070